10.95

UNEP

Radiation
Doses, Effects, Risks

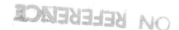

D1334900

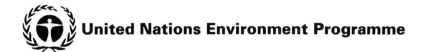 United Nations Environment Programme

Radiation
Doses, Effects, Risks

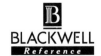

BLACKWELL
Reference

First edition published 1985

Blackwell Publishers
108 Cowley Road
Oxford OX4 1JF
UK

Three Cambridge Center
Cambridge, Massachusetts 02142
USA

British Library Cataloguing in Publication Data
Radiation : doses, effects, risks. – 2nd ed.
     I. United Nations Environment Programme
     613
     ISBN 0–631–18317–5

Library of Congress Cataloging-in-Publication Data
     Radiation : doses, effects, risks / United Nations Environment Programme.
     (Blackwell reference)
     ISBN 0–631–18317–5 (acid-free)
     1. Radiation–Health aspects.   2. Radiation–Environmental aspects. I. United Nations Environment Programme.
RA569.R26 1991   91–21298
618.9'897–dc20   CIP

ISBN 0–631–18317–5

DISCLAIMER
This booklet is largely based on the findings of the United Nations Scientific Committee on the Effects of Atomic Radiation, a subsidiary body of the United Nations General Assembly, and is edited by Geoffrey Lean. The publication does not necessarily reflect the views of the Committee, of the United Nations Environment Programme or of the editor.

Designed by Banson   Typeset in 9 on 13 pt Palatino
Printed in Great Britain at the Alden Press, Oxford
This book is printed on acid-free paper

Contents

CHAPTER ONE

INTRODUCTION

Few scientific issues arouse so much public controversy as the effects of radiation. Scarcely a week goes by in western developed countries without some expression of public feeling – and such developing countries as choose to have and advance nuclear programmes may well have the same experience. The disastrous nuclear accident at Chernobyl has greatly heightened public concern, and there is little sign that the radiation debate will die down in the near future.

Unfortunately, providing unbiased factual information to the public often takes second place to propagating opinions. Too often, anti-nuclear activists rely on emotion; too often, nuclear advocates rely on bland reassurance.

The United Nations Scientific Committee on the Effects of Atomic Radiation (UNSCEAR) collects available evidence on the sources and effects of radiation, and evaluates it. It considers the wide range of natural and man-made sources and estimates the risks from radiation exposures.

The effects of radiation are most evident at high doses, when cells may be killed and tissues severely damaged. At all doses, but at later times following exposure, radiation can cause cancers and induce genetic defects that can affect the children, grandchildren and later descendants of those irradiated.

The most important sources of radiation to the general public are not necessarily those that attract the greatest attention. Natural sources contribute most exposure. Nuclear power contributes only a small proportion of the radiation resulting from human activities; much less controversial activities such as the use of x-rays in medicine provide much greater doses. And everyday activities like burning coal, air travel and living in well-insulated homes in particular areas can substantially increase exposure to natural radiation. The greatest causes for concern and the greatest scope for reducing human exposure to radiation lie in some of these relatively uncontroversial pursuits.

INTRODUCTION

This booklet does not pretend to have all the answers. Our knowledge is still inadequate, even though more is known about the sources, effects and risks of radiation than about those of almost any other toxic agent. But the booklet does try to summarize what solid information there is so as to guide the debate onto firmer ground.

UNSCEAR was set up by the UN General Assembly in 1955 to evaluate doses, effects and risks from radiation on a worldwide scale. It brings together leading scientists from 21 member countries and is one of the most authoritative bodies of its kind in the world. It does not set, or even recommend, safety standards; rather it provides information on radiation which enables such bodies as the International Commission on Radiological Protection and national authorities to do so. Every few years it produces major reports assessing, in considerable detail, the doses, effects and risks from all sources of radiation to which man is exposed. This booklet is an attempt to summarize the most up-to-date material from the reports for the general reader. But it is no substitute for the reports themselves.

The next four chapters are based on UNSCEAR's most recent reports to the UN General Assembly: they have however not been reviewed or approved by the Committee. The last chapter is an attempt to discuss some general issues about the acceptability of risks from radiation, which are not part of the Committee's remit, and have not yet been considered in its reports.

CHAPTER TWO

RADIATION AND LIFE

There is nothing new about radioactivity except the uses to which people have been learning to put it. Both radioactivity and the radiation it produces existed on earth long before life emerged. Indeed they were present in space long before the earth itself appeared.

Radiation took part in the big bang which, as far as we know, gave birth to the universe about 20 billion years ago. Since then it has pervaded the cosmos. Radioactive materials became part of the earth at its very formation. Even man himself is slightly radioactive, for all living tissue contains traces of radioactive substances. But it is less than a century since humanity first discovered this elemental, universal phenomenon.

In 1896 Henri Becquerel, a French scientist, put some photographic plates away in a drawer with bits of a mineral containing uranium. When he developed them he found, to his surprise, that they had been affected by radiation. Soon afterwards, a young Polish-born chemist, Marie Curie, took the research further and was the first to coin the word "radioactivity". In 1898 she and her husband, Pierre, discovered that, as uranium gave off radiation, it mysteriously turned into other elements, one of which they called polonium, after her homeland, and another, radium, the "shining" element. Both Becquerel's and the Curies' work was greatly assisted by an earlier scientific breakthrough, when, in 1895 – and also by chance – Wilhelm Roentgen, a German physicist, discovered x-rays.

It was not long before Becquerel experienced the most troublesome drawback of radiation, the effect it can have on living tissues. He put a vial of radium in his pocket and damaged his skin. Marie Curie was to die of a malignant blood disease probably because of her exposure to radiation. At least 336 early radiation workers died from the doses they received, unaware of the need for protection.

Undeterred, a small group of brilliant, often young, scientists embarked on one of the most enthralling quests of all time, delving into the innermost secrets of matter itself. Their work was eventually to lead, in

RADIATION AND LIFE

1945, to the explosion of atomic bombs at the end of the Second World War with disastrous loss of life. It also led, in 1956, to the world's first sizeable nuclear power station, Calder Hall, in the United Kingdom. Meanwhile, ever since Roentgen's discoveries, there has been a continuous expansion of the medical uses of radiation.

The focus of the scientists' quest was the atom, and, more particularly, its structure. We now know that atoms behave like miniature solar systems; tiny nuclei are surrounded by orbiting "planets" called electrons. The nucleus is only about one hundred thousandth of the size of the entire atom, but it is so dense that it accounts for almost all its mass. It is generally a cluster of particles which cling tightly to each other.

Some of the particles carry a positive electrical charge and are called protons. The number of protons decide what element an atom belongs to; an atom of hydrogen has a single proton, an atom of oxygen eight, an atom of uranium 92. Each atom has the same number of orbiting electrons as it has protons; the electrons are negatively charged, and so they and the positively-charged protons balance each other. As a result, the atom as such is neither positive nor negative, but neutral.

The rest of the particles in the nuclear cluster are called neutrons because they carry no electrical charge. Atoms of the same element always have the same number of protons in their nuclei, but they can have varying numbers of neutrons. Those with different numbers of neutrons, but the same number of protons, belong to different varieties of the same element, and are called its "isotopes". These are distinguished by adding up the total numbers of particles in their nuclei. Thus uranium-238 has 92 protons and 146 neutrons; uranium-235 has the same 92 protons, but 143 neutrons. The atoms thus characterized are called "nuclides".

Some nuclides are stable, and lead uneventful, unchanging lives. But they are a minority. Most are unstable, and give vent to their instability by relentlessly trying to become something else. To take just one example, the particles in the nucleus of a uranium-238 atom are only just able to cluster together. Eventually a chunk of two protons and two neutrons – called an

THE DECAY OF URANIUM-238

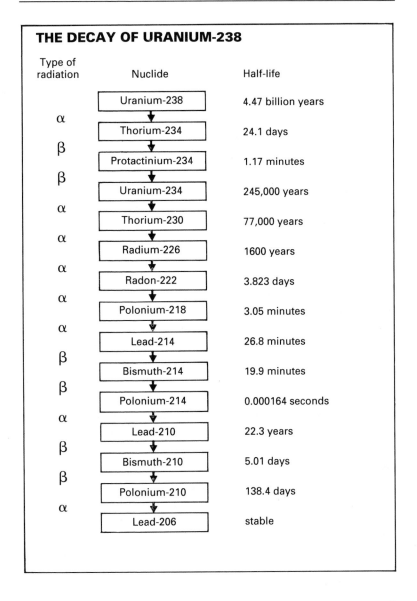

Type of radiation	Nuclide	Half-life
	Uranium-238	4.47 billion years
α	Thorium-234	24.1 days
β	Protactinium-234	1.17 minutes
β	Uranium-234	245,000 years
α	Thorium-230	77,000 years
α	Radium-226	1600 years
α	Radon-222	3.823 days
α	Polonium-218	3.05 minutes
α	Lead-214	26.8 minutes
β	Bismuth-214	19.9 minutes
β	Polonium-214	0.000164 seconds
α	Lead-210	22.3 years
β	Bismuth-210	5.01 days
β	Polonium-210	138.4 days
α	Lead-206	stable

"alpha" particle – will break away. As it goes, the uranium-238 turns into thorium-234 (with 90 protons and 144 neutrons). But thorium-234, too, is unstable; it, too, wants to become something else. It transforms itself by a different process; by emitting an electron – known as a "beta" particle – and substituting a neutron for a proton. It thus becomes protactinium-234, with 91 protons and 143 neutrons. This, in turn, is extremely unstable and loses no time in becoming uranium-234, and so the atom goes on shedding particles and transforming itself until it finally ends up as stable lead. Of course, there are many such sequences of transformation, or "decay" as it is called, with a large variety of patterns and combinations.

As each change takes place, energy is released, and is transmitted as radiation. The emission of two protons and two neutrons, as from uranium-238, is referred to as "alpha" radiation; the emission of an electron, as from thorium-234, is "beta" radiation. Frequently, the unstable nuclide will be so excited that the emission of particles is not sufficient to calm it down; it then gives off a vigorous burst of pure energy called "gamma" radiation. Like x-rays (which are similar in many ways), gamma radiation does not involve the emission of particles.

The whole transformation process is called "radioactivity", and the unstable nuclides "radionuclides". But while all radionuclides are unstable, some are more unstable than others. Protactinium-234, for example, can't wait to transform itself, while uranium-238 is extremely leisurely about the process. Half of a lump of protactinium-234 metamorphoses in little over a minute, whereas half a lump of uranium-238 will take four and a half billion years to turn into thorium-234. The period it takes half of any amount of an element to decay is known as its "half-life". The process goes on relentlessly. After one half-life 50 out of 100 atoms will have remained unchanged, during the next half-life 25 of these will decay, and so on exponentially. The number of transformations that take place each second in an amount of radioactive material is called its "activity". The activity is measured in units called becquerel, after the man who discovered the phenomenon; each becquerel equals one transformation a second.

RADIATION AND LIFE

The different forms of radiation are emitted with different energies and penetrating power – and so have different effects on living things. Alpha radiation, with its heavy chunk of neutrons and protons, is halted, for example, by a sheet of paper, and can scarcely penetrate the dead outer layers of the skin. So it is not dangerous unless substances emitting it are breathed in, eaten or get into the body through an open wound – but then it is especially damaging. Beta radiation is more penetrating. It will go through a centimetre or two of living tissue. Gamma radiation, which travels at the speed of light, is extremely penetrating and will go through anything short of a thick slab of lead or concrete.

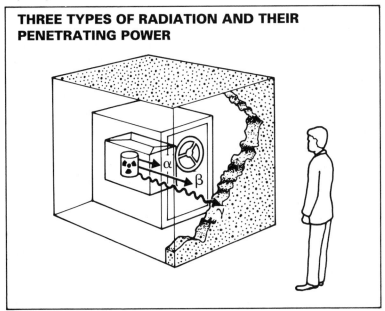

THREE TYPES OF RADIATION AND THEIR PENETRATING POWER

It is the energy of radiation which does the damage, and the amount of energy deposited in living tissue is called the "dose" – a rather misleading term originally intended to remind people of doses of medicines. The dose may come from any radionuclide, or number of

UNITS AND DOSES

Becquerel (Bq): The unit of activity. One becquerel corresponds to one disintegration per second of any radionuclide.

Gray (Gy): The unit of **absorbed dose**. One gray corresponds to one joule per kilogram.

Sievert (Sv): The unit of **equivalent dose and effective dose**. One sievert also corresponds to one joule per kilogram.

Absorbed dose: The quantity of energy imparted by ionizing radiation to a unit mass of material such as tissue.

Equivalent dose: Absorbed dose weighted for the potential of different radiations to do damage.

Effective dose: Equivalent dose weighted for the susceptibility to harm of different tissues in an individual.

Collective effective dose: Effective dose to a group of people from a source of radiation.

Collective effective dose commitment: Collective effective dose delivered over time to generations of people.

radionuclides, whether they remain outside the body or irradiate it from inside after being inhaled in air or swallowed in food or water. Doses are expressed in different ways depending on how much of the body, and what parts of it, are irradiated, whether one individual or many people are exposed, and the period during which the exposure takes place.

The amount of radiation energy that is absorbed per kilogram of tissue is called the absorbed dose and is expressed in units called gray (Gy). But this does not tell the full story because the same dose of alpha radiation is much more damaging than of beta or gamma radiation. So the

WEIGHTING FACTORS

Ovaries and testes	0.2
Red bone marrow	0.12
Colon	0.12
Lung	0.12
Stomach	0.12
Bladder	0.05
Breast	0.05
Liver	0.05
Oesophagus	0.05
Thyroid	0.05
Skin	0.01
Bone surface	0.01
Remainder	0.05
Whole body	1.00

Weighting factors recommended by the International Commission on Radiological Protection for the calculation of effective dose.

dose needs to be weighted for its potential to do damage, with alpha radiation given 20 times the weight of the others. This weighted dose is known as the "equivalent dose", and it is evaluated in units called sievert (Sv).

There is another refinement to be made. Some parts of the body are more vulnerable than others; a given equivalent dose of radiation is more likely to cause fatal cancer in the lung than in the thyroid, for example – and the reproductive organs are of particular concern because of the risk of genetic damage. The different parts of the body are therefore also given weightings. Once it has been weighted appropriately, the equivalent dose becomes the "effective dose", also expressed in sievert.

This, however, describes only individual doses. If you add up all the individual effective doses received by a group of people, the result is called the "collective effective dose", and this is expressed in man-sievert (man-Sv). But one further definition must be introduced, because many radionuclides decay so slowly that they are radioactive far into the future. This is the collective effective dose that will be delivered to generations of people over time, and it is called the "collective effective dose commitment".

This hierarchy of doses may appear complicated, but it does bring them into a coherent structure, and allows doses to be recorded consistently and comparably. To make things as simple as possible, the following chapters will avoid the use of these terms wherever possible. But frequently there is no alternative to them, to ensure accuracy and to eliminate ambiguity.

CHAPTER THREE

NATURAL SOURCES

By far the greatest part of the radiation received by the world's population comes from natural sources. Exposure to most of them is inescapable. Throughout the earth's history, radiation has fallen on its surface from outer space and risen from radioactive materials in its crust. People are irradiated in two ways. Radioactive substances in the environment may irradiate the body from the outside, or "externally". Or they may be inhaled in air or swallowed in food and water, and so irradiate people from inside, or "internally".

But though everyone on the planet receives natural radiation, some people get much more than others. This may result from where they live. Doses at some places, with particularly radioactive rocks or soils, are much higher than the average; at other places they are much less. Alternatively,

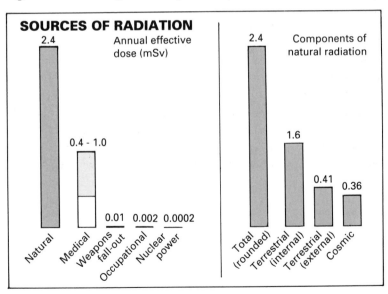

Average annual effective dose from natural and man-made sources.

it may result from their lifestyle. The use of particular building materials for houses, cooking with gas, open coal fires, home insulation, and even air travel all increase exposure to natural radiation.

Overall, terrestrial sources are responsible for most of man's exposure to natural radiation. In normal circumstances, they provide more than five-sixths of the annual effective doses received by individual people – most of it by internal irradiation. Cosmic rays contribute the remainder, mainly by external irradiation.

This chapter looks first at external radiation from cosmic and terrestrial sources. It then considers internal radiation, paying particular attention to radon, a radioactive gas which is the biggest single source of average doses from natural radiation. Finally, it turns to several practices, from coal burning to the use of fertilizers, which release radioactive substances from the ground and so enhance man's exposure to terrestrial sources.

EXTERNAL RADIATION
Cosmic rays

Just under half of man's exposure to external natural radiation comes from cosmic rays. Most of these originate from deep in interstellar space; some are released from the sun during solar flares. They irradiate the earth directly, and interact with the atmosphere to produce further types of radiation and different radioactive materials.

Nowhere escapes this universal, invisible shower. But it affects some parts of the globe more than others. The poles receive more than the equatorial regions, because the earth's magnetic field diverts the radiation. But, more important, the level increases with altitude, since there is less air overhead to act as a shield.

Someone living at sea-level will, on average, receive an effective dose of about 300 microsievert (millionths of a sievert) of cosmic radiation every year, but someone living above 2000 metres will receive several times as much. Air travel exposes passengers and crews to even higher dose rates,

NATURAL SOURCES

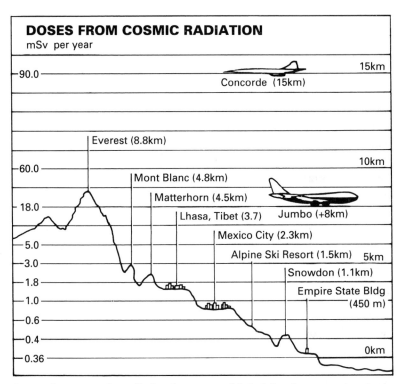

DOSES FROM COSMIC RADIATION
mSv per year

90.0	15km
	Concorde (15km)
60.0	Everest (8.8km)
	10km
18.0	Mont Blanc (4.8km)
	Matterhorn (4.5km)
	Lhasa, Tibet (3.7) Jumbo (+8km)
5.0	Mexico City (2.3km)
3.0	Alpine Ski Resort (1.5km) 5km
1.8	Snowdon (1.1km)
1.0	Empire State Bldg (450 m)
0.6	
0.4	0km
0.36	

Doses from cosmic radiation increase with height above sea level.

albeit for short periods at a time. Between 4000 metres, the altitude of the loftiest permanent Sherpa villages on the flanks of Mt Everest, and 12,000 metres, the level of the highest subsonic flights, exposures to cosmic radiation increase over 25 times. They rise further between 12,000 and 20,000 metres, the maximum altitude of supersonic aircraft.

A round trip from New York to Paris will expose a passenger to about 50 microsievert in a normal jet aeroplane, and about 20% less in a supersonic aircraft – although a supersonic aircraft is exposed to more intense radiation, it completes the journey much more quickly. Thus

13

---

someone living at sea-level could double his or her annual dose from cosmic radiation by taking six round trips across the Atlantic each year. In all, air travel results in a collective effective dose to the world's population of about 4000 man-sievert a year.

Terrestrial radiation

The main radioactive materials in rocks are potassium-40, rubidium-87, and two series of radioactive elements arising from the decay of uranium-238 and thorium-232, two long-lived radionuclides that have remained on earth since its origin.

Naturally, the levels of terrestrial radiation differ from place to place around the world, as the concentrations of these materials in the earth's crust vary. For most people, the variation is not particularly dramatic. Studies in France, Germany, Italy, Japan and the United States, for example, suggest that about 95% of the people live in areas where the average outdoor dose rate varies from 0.3 to 0.6 millisievert (thousandths of a sievert) a year. But some receive much greater doses; about 3% are exposed to one millisievert a year – half of them to over 1.4 millisievert a year. And there are places on earth where terrestrial radiation levels are very much higher still.

Near the city of Poços de Caldas, 200 kilometres north of São Paolo, Brazil, stands a small hill. Here researchers have discovered radiation dose rates up to about 800 times the average – 250 millisievert a year. As it happens, the hill is uninhabited. But only slightly less spectacular levels have been found in a coastal resort some 600 kilometres to the east.

Guarapari is a small town of 12,000 people, which every summer plays host to about 30,000 holiday makers. Particular spots on its beach have registered 175 millisievert a year. Radiation levels in the streets were found to be a good deal less, ranging from eight to 15 millisievert a year, but still many times higher than normal levels. It is much the same story in the fishing village of Meaipe, 50 kilometres to the south. Both stand on sands rich in thorium.

NATURAL SOURCES

Half a world away, on the southwest coast of India, 70,000 people live in a 55 kilometre long strip of land which also contains thorium-rich sands. Studies of 8513 people in the area showed that they absorbed, on average, 3.8 millisievert of radiation a year. Over 500 of them received more than 8.7 millisievert a year. About 60 absorbed more than 17 millisievert – over 40 times the average dose from external terrestrial radiation.

These areas in Brazil and India are the best studied hot-spots on earth. But levels of up to 400 millisievert a year have been found in Ramsar, Iran, where there are springs rich in radium. And other regions of high terrestrial natural radiation are known to exist in France, Madagascar and Nigeria.

UNSCEAR calculates that, on average, the world's people receive an effective dose of about 410 microsievert a year from external natural terrestrial radiation.

INTERNAL RADIATION

On average, two-thirds of the effective dose that people receive from natural sources comes from radioactive substances in the air they breathe, the food they eat and the water they drink.

Very little indeed of this internal dose comes from radioactive substances – like carbon-14 and tritium which are formed by cosmic radiation. Almost all of it is derived from terrestrial sources. On average, people receive about 180 microsievert a year from potassium-40, which is absorbed in the body along with non-radioactive potassium, an essential element. But by far the greatest amount comes from the elements resulting from the decay of uranium-238 – and, to a lesser extent, from the decay of thorium-232.

Some of these, like lead-210 and polonium-210, enter the body mainly in food. Both become concentrated in fish and shellfish; people eating large amounts of seafood can expect to receive correspondingly high doses.

Tens of thousands of people in the extreme north of the northern hemisphere subsist mainly on reindeer (or caribou) meat. The animals contain high concentrations of these two radioactive materials, particularly polonium-210, because during the winter they graze over large areas on lichen which accumulate them. The people end up with doses of polonium-210 up to 35 times normal levels.

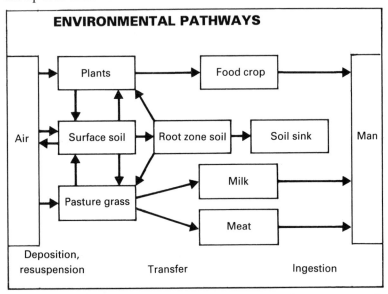

A typical set of pathways through the environment from a source of radiation in air.

Radioactive substances like these often take complex routes through the environment before reaching man. Such routes, or "pathways", are generally used to calculate doses received from particular sources.

Radon

The most important of all sources of natural radiation – it has recently been realized – is a tasteless, odourless, invisible, gas about eight times heavier than air, called radon. It has two main forms – radon-222, one of the radionuclides in the sequence formed by the decay of uranium-238, and radon-220, produced during the decay series of thorium-232. Radon-222 seems to be 20 times more important than radon-220, but for convenience both forms of the radioactive gas will be referred to here as "radon". Together with its "daughters", radionuclides formed as it decays, radon normally contributes about three-quarters of the annual internal effective dose received by individual people from terrestrial sources – and about half their doses from all natural sources put together. Most of the dose results from breathing in the radionuclides, particularly indoors, and most is contributed by the radon daughters rather than by the gas itself.

Radon seeps out of the earth all over the world, but levels in outside air vary markedly from place to place. Perhaps paradoxically, however, people are mainly exposed to radon indoors. In temperate parts of the

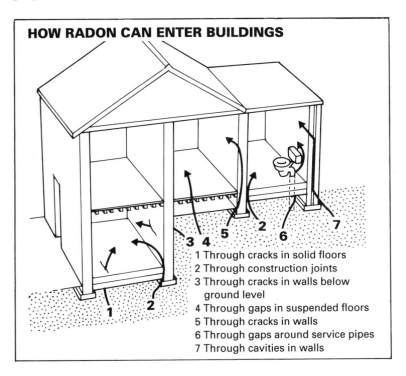

HOW RADON CAN ENTER BUILDINGS

1 Through cracks in solid floors
2 Through construction joints
3 Through cracks in walls below ground level
4 Through gaps in suspended floors
5 Through cracks in walls
6 Through gaps around service pipes
7 Through cavities in walls

NATURAL SOURCES

world the concentrations of radon indoors are, on average, about five to 10 times higher than they are outside. There are fewer measurements in tropical countries, but because buildings are kept much more open in the hotter climate, there is probably less difference between indoor and outdoor concentrations.

Radon concentrates in indoor air when buildings are, by and large, closed spaces. Once the gas gets in, mainly by filtering up through cellars and floors from the ground, or, to a lesser extent, by seeping out of the very materials used to build the edifice, it finds it hard to get out. Very high levels of radiation can result, especially if buildings happen to stand on particularly radioactive ground or have been constructed with especially radioactive materials. And tight-fitting doors and windows make it harder for the gas to escape.

Very high levels of radon are being found more and more frequently. In the late 1970s, concentrations of more of 10,000 becquerel per cubic metre, 2000 times typical levels in outside air, were found in homes in

Some typical activity concentrations of Radium-226.

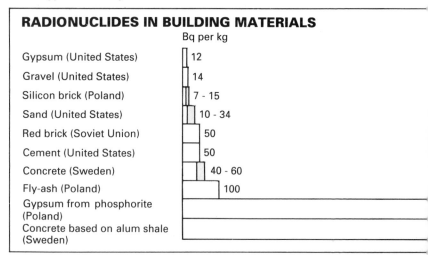

RADIONUCLIDES IN BUILDING MATERIALS
Bq per kg

Gypsum (United States)	12
Gravel (United States)	14
Silicon brick (Poland)	7 - 15
Sand (United States)	10 - 34
Red brick (Soviet Union)	50
Cement (United States)	50
Concrete (Sweden)	40 - 60
Fly-ash (Poland)	100
Gypsum from phosphorite (Poland)	
Concrete based on alum shale (Sweden)	

NATURAL SOURCES

Sweden and Finland. Since then, similar levels have been discovered in houses in the United Kingdom and the United States and other countries. As the number of homes examined has increased, so has the number found to contain such extreme concentrations.

In many countries, radon in homes is the largest single source of chronic exposure to radiation. In some cases, people have been found to be exposed to eight times the limit set for uranium miners – and they are usually unaware of the danger.

The commonest building materials – wood, bricks, and concrete – give off relatively little radon. Granite is much more radioactive and so is pumice stone, used, for example in the Soviet Union and Germany. And some materials have given builders, scientists – and residents – unwelcome surprises by proving to be especially radioactive.

For several decades, for example, alum shales were used in the making of concrete in Sweden which was incorporated in 350,000 to 700,000 Swedish homes. Then it was found that the shales were highly

580 - 740

1500

NATURAL SOURCES

radioactive. Their use was cut back and then stopped completely. Likewise, calcium silicate slag – a highly-radioactive by-product of the processing of phosphate ore – is used to make concrete and other building materials in North America. It has turned up in buildings in Idaho, Florida and Canada.

Phosphogypsum, another by-product from a different way of processing phosphate ore, has been widely used to make building blocks, plasterboard, partition systems and cement. It costs less than natural gypsum and was welcomed by environmentalists because it is a waste product, and so its use preserves natural resources and reduces pollution. In Japan alone, one million tonnes of the material were used in the construction industry in 1974. But it is also many times more radioactive than the natural gypsum it replaces, and people who live in houses containing it can expect to be exposed to about 30% more radiation than those who do not. In all, it is estimated that the annual use gives rise to a collective effective dose commitment of about 300,000 man-sievert.

Other highly radioactive waste products used in building include red mud bricks from aluminium production; blast furnace slag from iron works; and fly ash from the burning of coal.

Even wastes from uranium mining have been used. Between 1952 and 1966, tailings from uranium mills were used as building materials and under houses, particularly in Grand Junction, Colorado. In Port Hope, Ontario, material from a radium recovery plant was used for construction. In both cases the national governments had to step in and take remedial action because of the radiation doses received by inhabitants.

Despite concern about building materials, the ground underneath houses is almost always a much greater source of radon. In some cases, houses have been built on old radioactive wastes, including uranium mine tailings in Colorado, alum shale tailings in Sweden, radium factory tailings in Australia, and reclaimed land from phosphate mining in Florida. But even in more normal circumstances most radiation comes up through the floor.

NATURAL SOURCES

The highest radon levels in Helsinki, Finland, more than 2000 times greater than typical levels in outside air, were found in homes where the only significant source can have been the ground on which they stood. Even in Sweden, with its difficulties arising from the use of alum shale, new research indicates that the greatest problem is radon emanating from the ground.

Radon concentrations in the upper storeys of high buildings tend to be lower than at the ground floor. A survey in Norway showed that

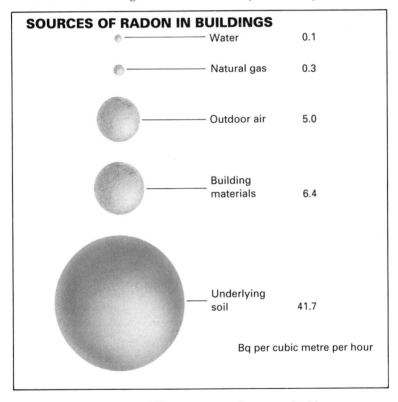

SOURCES OF RADON IN BUILDINGS

Water	0.1
Natural gas	0.3
Outdoor air	5.0
Building materials	6.4
Underlying soil	41.7

Bq per cubic metre per hour

Radon entry rates from different sources into a typical house.

wooden houses had higher radon concentrations than brick ones, despite the fact that the wood gave off virtually none of the gas: this was because the wood houses generally had fewer storeys and so their rooms were closer to the radon-emitting ground.

The integrity of the floorings of buildings determines how much of the radon rising up from the ground actually gets in. Studies of houses built on reclaimed phosphate land in Florida have demonstrated this; while in Chicago, houses with crawl spaces that were unpaved and open to the bare earth, were found to have radon concentrations well over 40 times typical outdoor levels, even though the concentrations in the soil were normal.

Radon levels in houses can be reduced by sealing floors and walls. By far the most effective way to reduce levels is to use fans to ventilate crawl spaces, because most radon gets in through the floor.

Water and natural gas provide further, if less important, sources of radon in homes. Usually the amounts of radon in water are extremely small, but some supplies, especially from deep wells, have very high concentrations. Such high levels have been found, for example, in wells in Finland and the United States, which supply water to Helsinki and, perhaps appropriately, Hot Springs, Arkansas, among other places. The most radioactive water supplies have radon activity concentrations of 100 million becquerel per cubic metre, the least, virtually nothing. In all, UNSCEAR estimates that less than 1% of the world's population consumes water containing more than a million becquerel of radon activity per cubic metre, and less than 10% drink water with over 100,000 becquerel per cubic metre.

Consuming water containing radon is not the main problem, even where levels are high. Generally, people take in most of their water in food and in hot drinks like tea and coffee. Boiling water and cooking with it releases most of the radon, and so the main intake comes from drinking the water cold. And even this is eliminated from the body very quickly.

People are more at risk from breathing in the radionuclides emitted by radon-rich water – particularly in the bathroom. A survey in Finnish

NATURAL SOURCES

RADON IN DIFFERENT ROOMS

Average radon concentrations (Bq per cubic metre)

Living room ▯ 200

Kitchen [   ] 3000

Bathroom [   ] 8500

homes showed that, on average, radon concentrations in bathrooms were about three times higher than in kitchens, where less water was used, and some 40 times higher than in living rooms. Meanwhile, a study in Canada showed that the amount of radon and its daughters in bathroom air increased rapidly during a seven minute warm shower, and that it was well over an hour and a half after the shower was turned off before levels returned to anything like what they were originally.

Radon also gets into "natural gas" in the ground. Processing and storage removes most of it before the gas reaches the consumer, but radon concentrations in homes can still increase significantly if the gas is burned in unvented stoves, heaters and other appliances. If the appliances are vented outside the house, the increase is negligible.

Much of the radon removed from natural gas during processing ends up in liquefied petroleum gas (LPG), which is produced as a by-product. But natural gas provides 10 to 100 times more radiation to homes on a national basis than the more radioactive LPG because much more of it is burned.

Energy conservation measures can greatly increase radon concentrations. Insulating houses and stopping draughts reduces ventilation. This conserves heat, but also allows radon to build up.

Sweden, where houses are particularly tightly sealed, is especially

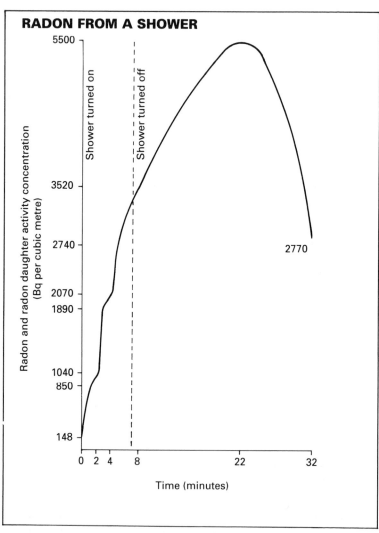

RADON FROM A SHOWER

Measurements taken in a shower room. The radon concentration in the water was **4400 becquerel per cubic metre.**

affected. For many years radon in homes was not thought to be a problem in Sweden, despite the use of alum shales; a survey in 1956 suggested that there were no grounds for serious concern at the ventilation rates of the time. But since the early 1950s, ventilation rates in Swedish houses have been steadily dropping in a drive to save energy. Between 1950 and the mid 1970s, ventilation rates were cut by more than half – and radon concentrations more than trebled. It has been calculated that every gigawatt year of electricity saved by reduced ventilation will expose Swedes to 5600 man-sievert of extra radiation.

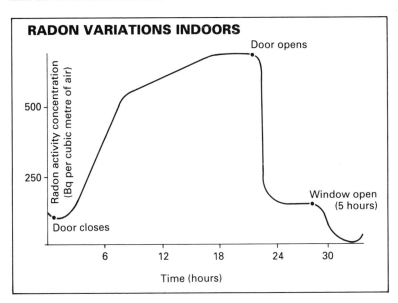

How radon concentrations varied in one apartment house over a 30 hour period.

Tight fitting windows and doors, high radon emissions from the ground to low rise buildings, and the use of alum shales in construction explain the Swedish situation. Information from other countries suggests that 90% of their houses have radon daughter activity concentrations under 50 becquerel per cubic metre, about 10 times typical outdoor levels, and no more than a few per cent contain amounts over 100 becquerel per cubic metre. In Sweden by contrast, more than 30% of the buildings have been found to be above this higher level, and average concentrations were four times those in other temperate lands.

However, Sweden may not be as exceptional as was once thought.

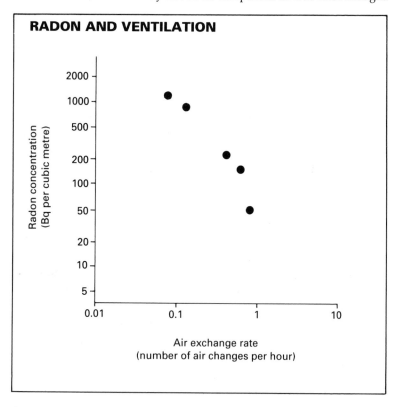

Average steady-state radon concentration in a residence as a function of ventilation rate.

NATURAL SOURCES

Other countries are beginning to find that their problems are greater than they suspected. It may be that part of the reason why Sweden appears to have a worse problem than elsewhere is that it carried out more extensive surveys earlier than in other countries.

The proportion of houses with radon daughter activity concentration levels between 1000 and 10,000 becquerel per cubic metre ranges from 0.01 to 0.1% in different countries. This means that quite large numbers of people may be exposed to high concentrations in their homes. Nevertheless, in countries with problems less acute than Sweden, three-quarters of the total collective equivalent dose will be accounted for by the homes with concentrations below 100 becquerel per cubic metre.

In its last report, UNSCEAR more than trebled its estimate of average indoor concentrations in temperate countries to over 50 becquerel per cubic metre; the tentative estimate for tropical countries is 15 becquerel per cubic metre. Over the world as a whole, the total effective dose due to exposure to radon and its daughters is normally about 1.2 millisievert a year – or about a half of the total estimated dose from all natural sources of radiation.

OTHER SOURCES

Coal, like most natural materials, contains traces of primordial radionuclides. Burning releases these, once locked deep in the earth, into the environment where they can affect people.

Though concentrations may vary a hundredfold from seam to seam, most coal contains lesser amounts of radioactive materials than the average in the earth's crust. But when coal is burned, most of its mineral matter is fused into ash, and most of the radioactive substances are concentrated in the ash as well. Most of the ash is heavy and drops to the bottom of a power plant furnace. Lighter fly-ash, however, is carried up the chimney of the plant. How much comes out depends on how much of an attempt is made to stop it with anti-pollution devices.

The cloud from the chimneys irradiates people and the pollution also settles on the ground and contaminates food crops. Some of it may even get

NATURAL SOURCES

back into the air as dust. The production of each gigawatt year of electrical energy is estimated to lead to a total collective effective dose commitment of four man-sievert, which means that each year the world's coal power stations produce a collective effective dose commitment of 2000 man-sievert.

Less coal is used for cooking and heating in private homes, but a greater proportion of the ash escapes. So the world's stoves and fireplaces may well emit as much ash to the atmosphere as its power stations. Furthermore, unlike most power stations, private homes have low chimneys and are normally in the heart of population centres; so much more of the pollution will fall on people. Very little attention has been paid to this issue, but, at an extremely rough estimate, domestic cooking and heating with coal may produce an annual collective effective dose commitment in the range of 2000 to 40,000 man-sievert throughout the world.

Little, too, is known of the effect of the fly-ash collected by pollution control equipment. In some countries more than a third of it is re-used, mainly in cement and concrete. Some concretes are four-fifths fly-ash. It is also used in roadbuilding and to improve farm soil. All of these applications could lead to increased radiation exposures, but very little information has been published in this field.

Geothermal energy is another source of increased radiation. Several countries tap reservoirs of steam and hot water trapped in the earth to generate electricity or to heat buildings; one source has been powering turbines at Larderello in Italy since the turn of the century. Examination of the emissions of this and the Geysers power plant in the United States, along with two very much smaller Italian plants, suggests that they produce a collective effective dose commitment of two man-sievert per gigawatt year of electricity output – approximately half the corresponding dose produced by coal fired power stations. Geothermal energy accounts for only 0.1% of present world energy production, and so makes only a tiny contribution to the world's radiation exposure. But it may become much

COMPARISON OF COLLECTIVE DOSE COMMITMENTS

man sievert

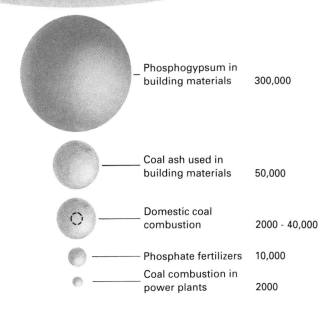

Natural background   12 million

Phosphogypsum in
building materials   300,000

Coal ash used in
building materials   50,000

Domestic coal
combustion   2000 - 40,000

Phosphate fertilizers 10,000

Coal combustion in
power plants   2000

Comparison of annual collective dose received directly from natural sources and the collective dose commitments from man's annual use of naturally radioactive materials.

more important in future, since many studies suggest that its potential is very great.

Phosphate rock is mined extensively around the world, mainly for use in fertilizers; about 130 million tonnes were produced in 1982. Most of the deposits of phosphate ore under exploitation contain high concentrations of uranium. Radon is released during mining and processing of the ores, and the fertilizers themselves are radioactive and

---

contaminate food. This contamination is normally only slight, but it may be greater if the fertilizer is applied to the soil in liquid form or if phosphate products are fed to animals. Such products are, indeed, widely used in livestock feed supplements and, when fed to dairy cattle, can significantly increase radium levels in milk. All these aspects of the phosphate industry give rise from annual use to a collective effective dose commitment of about 10,000 man-sievert.

CHAPTER FOUR

MAN-MADE SOURCES

Over the last few decades man has "artificially" produced several hundred radionuclides. And he has learned to use the power of the atom for a wide variety of purposes, from medicine to weapons, from the production of energy to the detection of fires, from illuminating watches to prospecting for minerals. All increase the radiation dose both to individual people and to mankind as a whole.

Individual doses from man-made sources of radiation vary greatly. Most people receive a relatively small amount of artificial radiation; but a few get many thousand times the amount they receive from natural sources.

This variability is generally greater for man-made sources than for natural ones. Most man-made sources, too, can be controlled more readily than most natural ones; though exposure to external radiation due to fall-out from past nuclear explosions, for example, is almost as inescapable and uncontrollable as that due to cosmic rays from beyond the atmosphere or to radiation from out of the earth itself.

MEDICAL SOURCES

At present, medicine is much the greatest source of human exposure from man-made radiation. Indeed in many countries it is responsible for nearly all of the dose received from artificial sources.

Radiation is used for both diagnosing and treating disease. X-ray machines are one of the most useful tools at the service of doctors – and new, sophisticated, diagnostic techniques using radioisotopes are spreading rapidly. Radiation treatment is also, paradoxically, one of the main ways of fighting cancer.

Obviously, individual doses vary enormously – from zero (for someone who has not even had an x-ray examination) to many thousand times the annual average dose from natural radiation (for some patients undergoing treatment for cancer). Yet there is remarkably little reliable and

MAN-MADE SOURCES

COLLECTIVE DOSE COMMITMENTS

Source	Annual collective dose (man Sv)
Natural background	12 million
Medical (diagnostic)	2 - 5 million
Occupational exposures	10,000
Nuclear power production	1000

Source	Collective dose commitment (man Sv)
Weapons fall-out from all test explosions	5 million
Nuclear accidents	600,000

The total collective dose commitments (over all time) are from atmospheric nuclear testing in the 1950s and 60s and from nuclear accidents (mostly Chernobyl).

representative information such as UNSCEAR needs to calculate doses to the world's population. Not enough is known about how many people are irradiated each year, or about what doses they receive to what parts of their bodies.

In principle, medical radiation is beneficial. But it does seem that people often receive doses that are unnecessarily high. These could be considerably reduced without any loss of efficiency. Since medical radiation accounts for such a high proportion of the exposure to man-made sources, the benefit of such reductions would also be great.

Diagnostic x-rays are much the commonest form of medical

MAN-MADE SOURCES

radiation. Worldwide, about 1400 million x-ray examinations are carried out every year; but three-quarters of them are received by the one-quarter of the world's people that inhabit developed countries while the 14% of the people that live in the countries with the least developed health care share only 2% of them. In most developing countries both equipment and examinations are concentrated in the cities and rarely reach the majority of people who live in rural areas. In many developing countries 30 to 70% of x-ray machines are out of order. Some authors point out that, in effect, about three-quarters of the world's population have no chance of receiving any radiological examination, no matter what disease they may have.

In most countries half of all medical x-ray examinations are of the chest. But mass chest x-rays are becoming less useful as the incidence of tuberculosis falls. What is more, there is now good evidence that early detection of lung cancer by these means does not significantly improve the prospect of survival. The frequency of these examinations has fallen heavily in many industrialized countries including Sweden, the United Kingdom, and the United States. In some other countries, however, a third of the people are still examined every year.

Over recent years there have been technical improvements which, if applied correctly, should reduce unnecessary doses to patients from x-ray examinations. Disappointingly, studies in Sweden and the United States show that they have resulted in little or no reduction in doses.

Doses vary widely from hospital to hospital even within the same country. Several studies in Germany, the United Kingdom, and the United States show that the doses delivered by the x-ray beam as it enters the body vary a hundredfold. Meanwhile, another survey has shown that the irradiated area is sometimes twice as large as it should be. Other studies indicate that many facilities produce poor x-ray pictures, and give unnecessary radiation exposure because their equipment performs badly.

Nevertheless, there are cases where radiation exposures have indeed fallen because of improved equipment and practice. In other cases, considerable gains in diagnostic efficiency have been made by deliberately

33

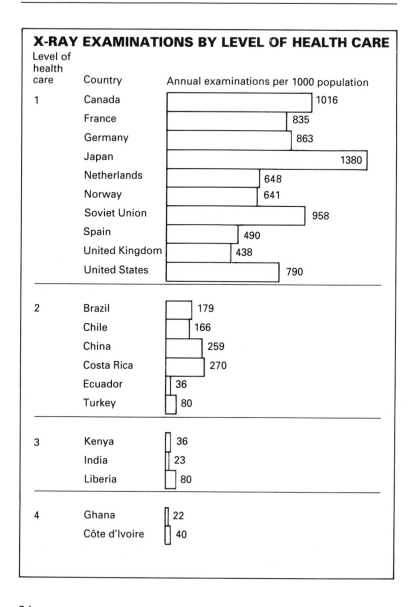

X-RAY EXAMINATIONS BY LEVEL OF HEALTH CARE

Level of health care	Country	Annual examinations per 1000 population
1	Canada	1016
	France	835
	Germany	863
	Japan	1380
	Netherlands	648
	Norway	641
	Soviet Union	958
	Spain	490
	United Kingdom	438
	United States	790
2	Brazil	179
	Chile	166
	China	259
	Costa Rica	270
	Ecuador	36
	Turkey	80
3	Kenya	36
	India	23
	Liberia	80
4	Ghana	22
	Côte d'Ivoire	40

MAN-MADE SOURCES

increasing doses by moderate amounts. The object must be to keep exposure to the lowest level that is necessary by improving techniques, instrumentation and practices, by carefully justifying procedures, and using alternatives to x-rays. Average doses per person could be cut in half in developed countries without jeopardizing the benefits of x-ray examinations.

Doses from dental x-rays do seem to have come down as a result of technical improvements. This is important, not least because these are the most frequent x-ray examinations in many industrialized countries. Limiting the x-ray beam more tightly, filtering it further to remove unnecessary radiation, using faster films, and adequate shielding all reduce exposure.

Breast examinations have also benefited from reduced doses. Mammographic techniques introduced in the second half of the 1970s generally give much lower doses than those delivered by earlier equipment, and it may be feasible to reduce them further without impairing the quality of the x-ray picture. This reduction has been matched by an increase in the number of breast examinations undertaken – they more than doubled in both Sweden and the United States between 1977 and 1979.

The use of another new technique, computed tomography, is rapidly increasing – it rose a hundredfold in Sweden between 1973 and 1979. It is considered to be the greatest improvement in the use of radiation for diagnosis since Roentgen's discovery of x-rays, but may lead, in some instances, to higher radiation doses to the patient.

Working out the average doses received by large numbers of people is extremely difficult, partly because data on the frequency of x-ray examinations are so limited – particularly from some of the developing

This table shows the number of diagnostic x-ray examinations per 1000 population in countries arranged according to levels of health care. The figures are from UNSCEAR's 1988 report and are the latest available for each country, ranging from the 1970s to the 1980s.

MEAN DOSES FROM VARIOUS X-RAY EXAMINATIONS

millisievert

Examination	China	France	Italy	Japan	Soviet Union	United States
Skull		1.4	0.22	0.09	0.17	0.13
Cervical spine		1.4	0.14	0.30	0.23	0.20
Chest	0.21	0.28	0.18	0.05	0.36	0.07
Abdomen	4.5	2.6	1.9	0.29	1.5	0.56
Urogram		10.4	7.1	0.70	2.5	1.6
Pelvis and hip		1.6	3.2	0.25	1.5	0.6

The table shows that diagnostic x-ray examinations may be defined or performed differently in different countries, resulting in a range of doses. All figures are from the early 1980s.

countries. Good data on the frequency of examinations and absorbed doses are available predominantly from developed countries, containing a quarter of the worlds' people. Fragmentary data are available for countries containing another quarter of the world's people – but none at all from the nations that are home to the other half. The wide variation in doses from hospital to hospital complicates matters further, because it means that data from one clinic usually cannot be taken to be representative.

Until recently, attempts to assess the average population dose from x-ray examinations have been limited to trying to determine that which may entail genetic consequences. It is called the genetically significant dose, or GSD. Its magnitude depends heavily on two factors. One is whether the patients are likely subsequently to have children; this is heavily influenced by their age. The other is the dose the x-rays deliver to the reproductive

MAN-MADE SOURCES

germ cells. This is linked to the type of examinations carried out; in the United Kingdom the biggest contributors to the GSD in 1977 were examinations of the pelvis and lower back, of the upper femur and hip, of the bladder and urinary tract, and barium enemas.

The GSD in the United Kingdom that year was estimated at about 0.12 millisievert. It was about 0.15 millisievert in Japan in 1979, 0.22 in the United States in 1980, and 0.25 in Italy in 1983. It has topped 0.40 in Sweden, Puerto Rico and Germany.

Since 1982, UNSCEAR has attempted to go further and work out the effective dose for patients, to assess the potential harm to other tissues in the body beside the reproductive organs. This is difficult to do, even in principle, because the usual means of calculating this dose is not well suited to medical exposures. There are also technical difficulties. Estimating the effective dose requires accurate data on how much radiation has been absorbed by up to a dozen different organs or tissues for each examination. The distribution of these doses can differ a thousandfold or more for the same type of x-ray examination – despite technical advances that were actually expected to reduce such variations.

Radioisotopes are used to explore many bodily processes and locate tumours. Their use has increased rapidly over the last 30 years, but they are still far less frequent than x-ray examinations. Information is scanty, but what exists suggests that the annual number of examinations ranges from seven to 49 examinations per 1000 inhabitants in industrialized countries, and less than one per 1000 inhabitants in developing ones. Annual effective doses per person range almost tenfold in developed countries, from 0.017 millisievert in the United Kingdom to 0.14 millisievert in the United States, with very much lower doses in developing nations.

Some 18,000 radiotherapy machines in use worldwide treat approximately 5 million patients every year, combating cancer by heavily irradiating malignant tissues to try to kill tumour cells. Yet again, there is very limited information about how much they are used, or what exposures populations receive. There are also worrying variations in dose: even in

MAN-MADE SOURCES

highly industrialized countries 15% of the institutions tested by the World Health Organization and the International Atomic Energy Agency made errors of over 10% in dosimetry. The actual doses given to each patient are high but they are usually given to people with a relatively short life expectancy and little likelihood of having children. They are also given to comparatively few people and so make a very small contribution to the overall dose: the annual genetically significant dose ranges from 0.015 millisievert in the most industrialized nations to 0.0003 millisievert in the least developed countries.

The hundreds of millions of small doses given in x-ray examinations each year far outweigh the relatively few high doses given to cancer patients; indeed they comprise 90 to 95% of the total dose. The average effective dose from all medical exposures per inhabitant of industrialized countries may be around one millisievert a year – about half the average dose from natural sources. This estimate conceals wide variations; it may even vary threefold from country to country. It is harder to calculate worldwide doses, since there is so little information about developing countries.

In 1982, UNSCEAR estimated that developing countries brought the world average down to about 0.4 millisievert per person per year, but it now thinks that this may be much too low. Although there are far fewer x-ray examinations in developing countries, they may deliver doses 10 to 20 times higher than in industrialized nations. Many machines seriously malfunction, giving high exposures. There is a widespread use of fluoroscopy, which can give 15 times the dose of conventional radiography. So UNSCEAR now believes that the population of developing countries may receive as high an average dose as the people of industrialized nations. So the worldwide average could be as high as one millisievert per person per year.

On this basis, UNSCEAR has worked out upper and lower estimates

This table summarizes some of the ways listed in UNSCEAR's 1988 report that x-ray doses can be reduced.

PROCEDURES TO REDUCE DOSES IN X-RAY EXAMINATIONS

Examination	Procedure	Entrance dose reduction factor
All types	Elimination of medically unnecessary procedures	1.2
	Introduction of quality assurance programme (QA)	2
Radiography	Decrease in rejected films through QA programme	1.1
	Increase of peak kilovoltage	1.5
	Beam collimation	1 - 3
	Use of rare earth screens	2 - 4
	Increase of filtration	1.7
	Change from photofluorography to chest radiography	4 - 10
	Use of carbon fibre materials	2
	Gonadal shielding	2 - 10
Pelvimetry	Use of CT topogram	5 - 10
Fluoroscopy	Use of 105 mm camera	4 - 5
	Radiologist technique	2 - 10
	Variable aperture iris on TV camera	3
	Change from chest fluoroscopy to radiography	20
Digital radiography	Decrease in contrast resolution	2 - 3
	Use of pulsed system	2
Mammography	Intensifying screens	2 - 5
	Optimal compression	1.3 - 1.5
	Filtration	3

for worldwide collective doses. The lower, which assumes that the same average doses are delivered by examinations in countries with differing levels of health care, suggests a collective effective dose of 1.8 million man-sievert a year. The upper estimate, assuming that absorbed doses are 10 to 20 times higher in developing countries, indicates a collective effective dose of 5 million man-sievert a year. The collective doses will increase as the world's population grows and ages and as more people come to live in cities; it will probably increase by 50% by the year 2000 and could more than double in another quarter of a century.

NUCLEAR EXPLOSIONS

For the last 40 years, everyone has been exposed to radiation from fall-out from nuclear weapons. Virtually none of this comes from the bombs actually

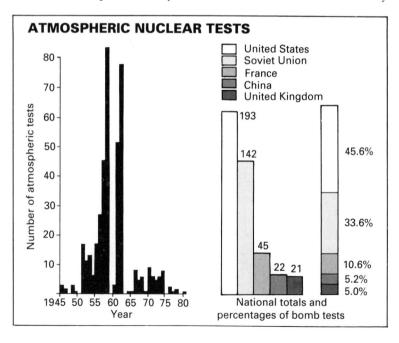

ATMOSPHERIC NUCLEAR TESTS

United States
Soviet Union
France
China
United Kingdom

Number of atmospheric tests

193
142
45
22 21

45.6%
33.6%
10.6%
5.2%
5.0%

National totals and
percentages of bomb tests

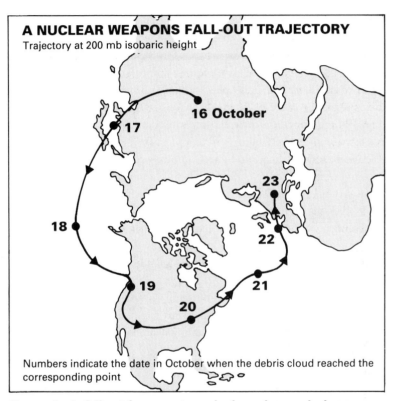

A NUCLEAR WEAPONS FALL-OUT TRAJECTORY
Trajectory at 200 mb isobaric height

16 October

17

18

23

22

21

19

20

Numbers indicate the date in October when the debris cloud reached the corresponding point

Tropospheric fall-out from an atmospheric nuclear explosion on 16 October, 1980. Only one of several trajectories traced at different isobaric heights is shown.

dropped on Hiroshima and Nagasaki in 1945; almost all is the result of atmospheric nuclear explosions carried out to test nuclear weapons.

This testing reached two peaks; the first between 1954 and 1958 when the United States, the Soviet Union and the United Kingdom were all exploding devices; the second, and greater, in 1961 and 1962 when the United States and the Soviet Union were the main contributors. During the first period, United States tests dominated – during the second, tests by the Soviet Union.

In 1963 the three countries signed the Partial Test Ban Treaty, undertaking not to test nuclear weapons in the atmosphere, oceans, and outer space. Over the next two decades France and China conducted a series of much smaller atmospheric tests with declining frequency, but they, too, stopped after 1980 and there have been no atmospheric tests since then. Underground tests are still being carried out, but they generally give rise to virtually no fall-out.

Some of the radioactive debris from atmospheric tests lands relatively close to the site of the explosion. Some stays in the troposphere, the lowest layer of the atmosphere, and is carried by the wind around the world at much the same latitude; as it travels it gradually falls to earth, remaining, on average, about a month in the air. But most is pushed into the stratosphere, the next layer of the atmosphere (from about 10 to 50 kilometres up) where it stays for many months, and whence it slowly descends all over the earth.

These various types of fall-out contain several hundred different radionuclides, but only a few contribute much to human exposure, as most are produced in very small amounts or decay quickly. Only four contribute more than 1% to the collective effective dose commitment of the world population from nuclear explosions. These are, in declining order of importance, carbon-14, caesium-137, zirconium-95 and strontium-90.

The doses from these, and other radionuclides, are delivered over different periods, because they decay at different rates. Zirconium-95, which has a half-life of 64 days, has already delivered practically all its dose. Caesium-137 and strontium-90 both have half-lives of about 30 years, and so will have delivered most of their doses by the end of the century. Only carbon-14, with its 5730 year half-life, will stay active into the far future, though at low dose rates; by the year 2000 it will have delivered only 7% of its eventual contribution.

Annual doses have closely followed testing, peaking in 1958 and, especially, in 1963-4. In 1963 the average annual doses amounted to about

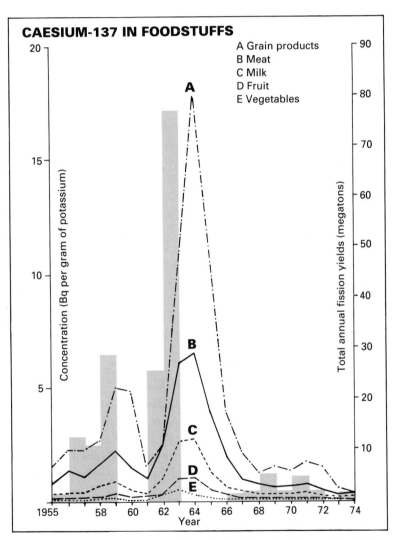

Variation of caesium-137 in various Danish foods. The yearly yield from atmospheric nuclear tests is shown for comparison.

7% of the equivalent exposure to natural radiation; this decreased to 2% by 1966, and 1% by the early 1980s. If no more atmospheric tests take place future annual doses will get smaller and smaller.

These averages do conceal considerable variations. The northern hemisphere, where most of the testing has taken place, has also received most of the fall-out. Reindeer herders in the extreme north accumulate doses of caesium-137 of between 100 and 1000 times average levels just as they receive more natural radiation; like natural polonium-210, the caesium sticks to the surface of the lichens and concentrates in the lichen-reindeer food chain. Some people in the vicinity of test sites, such as some inhabitants of the Marshall Islands, and a boatload of Japanese fishermen who happened to pass nearby, have received high doses.

The total collective effective dose commitment from atmospheric nuclear explosions conducted so far amounts to 30 million man-sievert. Only 12% of this had been delivered by 1980, the rest will reach man over thousands of years.

NUCLEAR POWER

The production of nuclear power is much the most controversial of all the man-made sources of radiation, yet it makes a very small contribution to human exposure. In normal operation, most discharges from nuclear facilities emit very little radiation to the environment.

By the end of 1988 there were 429 nuclear power reactors in operation in 25 countries, worldwide. They produced about 17% of the world's electricity from a total generating capacity of 311 gigawatts. Capacity had doubled in little over five years, and quadrupled in 10, but future growth rates are unclear. The International Atomic Energy Agency forecast in 1987 that there would be a worldwide capacity of 400 to 500 gigawatts of electricity in the year 2000.

These power stations are just part of the nuclear fuel cycle. This starts with the mining and milling of uranium ore, and proceeds to the making of nuclear fuel. After use in power stations the irradiated fuel is sometimes

MAN-MADE SOURCES

"reprocessed" to recover uranium and plutonium. Eventually the cycle will end with the disposal of nuclear wastes.

At each stage in this cycle radioactive materials are released. UNSCEAR has set out to evaluate the doses delivered to the public at each part of the cycle both in the short term and over many hundreds of years. This is a complicated and difficult undertaking. For a start, emissions vary widely, even from similar installations; the levels of radioactive gases given off by boiling water reactors (BWRs), for example, can vary more than a millionfold from plant to plant and year to year.

The doses also vary over space and time. Generally speaking, the further people live from a particular nuclear installation the less radiation they will receive from it; and whereas some installations are in remote areas, others are near centres of population. These installations emit a variety of radionuclides which decay at different rates; most are of only local importance because they decay rapidly; some live long enough to spread right around the world; and some remain in the environment virtually for ever. Different radionuclides also behave differently in the environment; some spread quickly, others move very little.

To get to grips with this confusing situation, UNSCEAR has developed hypothetical model installations, designed to be typical facilities, in typical geographical areas, surrounded by typical population densities. It has also studied information on discharges from the world's nuclear plants and produced average releases for each gigawatt year of electricity generated. These generalizations give an idea of the overall impact of the nuclear power programme but, obviously, cannot be applied indiscriminately to any individual plant. They must be treated with the utmost caution; they cannot be taken at face value, and are subject to a large number of assumptions spelled out in the UNSCEAR reports.

About half the world's uranium ore comes from open-cast mines, and half from underground ones. It is then taken to mills, usually nearby, for processing. Both mines and mills give off radioactive discharges to the environment. The mines account for nearly all the combined dose from the

NUCLEAR POWER AND NUMBER OF REACTORS 1989

Nuclear electricity as % of total supplied

Country		%	Number of reactors
France		75%	64
Belgium		61%	7
Rep. of Korea		50%	11
Hungary		50%	4
Sweden		45%	12
Switzerland		42%	5
Spain		38%	10
Finland		35%	4
Taiwan		35%	6
Bulgaria		33%	7
Germany		30%	36
Japan		28%	51
Czechoslovakia		28%	16
United Kingdom		22%	40
United States		19%	114
Canada		16%	22
Soviet Union		12%	72
Argentina		11%	3
South Africa		7%	2
Yugoslavia		6%	1
Netherlands		5%	2
India		2%	14
Brazil		0.7%	2
Pakistan		0.2%	1
Mexico		na	2
Italy*		0%	2
China		0%	3
Cuba		0%	2
Iran		0%	2
Romania		0%	5

* Neither reactor in Italy generates electricity

MAN-MADE SOURCES

two operations in the short term. But the mills are responsible for a much greater long-term problem; they produce large amounts of waste, or "tailings" – more than 120 million tonnes are already stored at active mill sites, mainly in North America. If current trends continue, there will be 500 million tonnes by the end of the century.

The wastes remain radioactive millions of years after mills cease operation, providing potentially the greatest long-term contribution to human exposure from nuclear power, albeit resulting in radiation exposures that are a very small fraction of natural background exposures. But this contribution could be reduced greatly, at least in the short term. At present, tailings tend to be kept in open, uncontained piles, or are covered with water behind dams and dikes. Providing better protection can cut radioactive emissions by up to a millionfold: open pile tailings can, for example, be covered with asphalt or polyvinylchloride, though such covers must be well-maintained.

After leaving the mills, the uranium is turned into fuel by further processing and purification and, usually, by passing through an enrichment plant. These processes give rise to both airborne and liquid discharges, but the doses are very much smaller than from other parts of the fuel cycle.

The fuel is now ready to be used in reactors to produce power. There are five main kinds of reactor in operation; pressurized water reactors and boiling water reactors (PWR, BWR), which were originally developed in the United States and are now the commonest types in the world; gas-cooled reactors (GCR), developed, and predominantly used, by the United Kingdom and France; pressurized heavy water reactors (PHWR), largely confined to Canada; and light-water cooled graphite moderated reactors (LWGR), which are in operation only in the Soviet Union. Besides these, there are a few fast breeder reactors, which have been envisaged as the next

Countries with nuclear reactors in operation and under construction and the percentage of each country's electricity generated by nuclear reactors.

generation of nuclear power plants in Europe, Japan and the Soviet Union.

The quantities of different types of radioactive materials released from these reactors vary widely, not only from type to type, not only between different designs within these types, but even between reactors of the same design. They also vary from year to year for the same reactor, partly because the amount of maintenance work (which gives rise to the

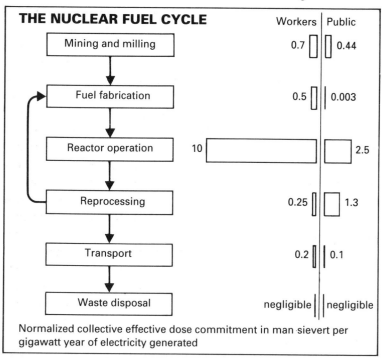

THE NUCLEAR FUEL CYCLE

	Workers	Public
Mining and milling	0.7	0.44
Fuel fabrication	0.5	0.003
Reactor operation	10	2.5
Reprocessing	0.25	1.3
Transport	0.2	0.1
Waste disposal	negligible	negligible

Normalized collective effective dose commitment in man sievert per gigawatt year of electricity generated

Radiation exposures to nuclear workers and the public, expressed in terms of collective dose per gigawatt year of electricity generated.

greatest routine discharges) differs each year.

Recently releases from reactors have tended to decrease despite the increasing electrical output of plants. This is partly due to technological

---

improvements, and partly due to stricter radiation protection measures.

After use in power stations, about 5% of the world's irradiated fuel is reprocessed to remove uranium and plutonium for re-use. Six countries currently have their spent fuel reprocessed and another seven are contracted to do so, five are considering burying their spent fuel unreprocessed, and the rest are uncommitted. However, only three commercial reprocessing plants are now operating: at Marcoule and La Hague in France, and at Sellafield (formerly Windscale) in the United Kingdom. The releases from Marcoule are particularly tightly controlled and are the lowest because it discharges to the river Rhône. The other two plants discharge into the sea, adding very small amounts to local average natural background levels. Discharges from the two plants are now similar.

Low-level wastes are normally disposed of by shallow burial. Facilities range from simple trenches or pits covered with soil, to concrete structures containing treated wastes and covered with materials that provide proper protection against the weather. Some short-lived intermediate level wastes are also disposed of in this way. Between 1949 and 1982, when a temporary moratorium was imposed, 142,000 tonnes of low-level wastes were dumped at sea. No disposal of highly radioactive wastes from nuclear power production – the last stage in the fuel cycle – has yet taken place. National authorities have been storing them and most of the intermediate level wastes. Much work has been done on the immobilization of high and intermediate level wastes and on their ultimate disposal in stable geological formations on land, or on, or under, the seabed. Once disposal has taken place, virtually none of the radioactivity in the wastes is expected to reach man in the foreseeable future.

In all, UNSCEAR estimates, the operation of the fuel cycle contributes a short-term collective effective dose commitment of about four man-sievert for every gigawatt year of electricity produced by the world's nuclear reactors. Mining contributes 0.3 man-sievert; milling 0.04 man-sievert; mine and mill tailings 0.1 man-sievert; and fuel fabrication a mere 0.003 man-sievert. Nuclear reactors are responsible for the bulk of the dose,

MAN-MADE SOURCES

contributing about 2.5 man-sievert. Transport of radioactive materials adds 0.1 man-sievert and reprocessing accounts for another 1.3 man-sievert.

Of this short-term dose, 90% is delivered within a year of the discharge of the radioactive materials – 98% within five years. Almost all of it is received by the local and regional populations, people living within a few thousand kilometres of the installations.

But the fuel cycle operations also give off longer-lived radionuclides which become distributed around the globe. UNSCEAR estimates the collective effective dose commitment from this source as 60 man-sievert for every gigawatt year of electricity produced, of which 10%, or six man-sievert, will be delivered during the first 100 years. This is similar to the collective dose received over the same period by the regional and local inhabitants, but since the collective dose is spread over far more people, individual doses are very much lower, and are a minute fraction of natural background doses. The remaining 90% of the global collective dose, delivered between 100 and several million years after the releases, will result in even smaller doses.

These figures do not include doses contributed by nuclear waste. The effect of waste disposal is thought to be negligible over the next few thousand years, and only 0.1 to 1% of the total dose commitment from nuclear power thereafter. The total collective effective dose commitment from long-lived radionuclides is some 200 man-sievert for every gigawatt year of electricity produced over the next 10,000 years. But these estimates are necessarily very uncertain. There are great difficulties in making them, not least in predicting future waste management techniques and practices, population sizes and habits over this time scale. So UNSCEAR warns against using these figures in decision-making and suggests that little significance should be attributed to them.

The annual collective effective dose caused by the nuclear fuel cycle is about 800 man-sievert. This is about 10,000 times less than the annual collective effective dose from natural radiation.

People living near nuclear installations do, of course, receive higher doses than the average. Even so, typical doses around nuclear reactors at present range between a fraction of 1% and a few per cent of doses from natural sources. Meanwhile, the dose received even by people most at risk around Sellafield from the 1985 releases of caesium-137 was probably under a quarter of what they received from natural radiation in the same year, and current levels are even lower.

All the above figures, of course, assume that the nuclear plants operate normally; for very much larger quantities of nuclear materials may be released in accidents.

ACCIDENTS

As in any human activity, accidents inevitably happen in the handling of nuclear materials. Between 1944 and 1987, 284 nuclear accidents were recorded around the world, apart from the Chernobyl disaster: 1358 people were affected, of whom 33 died. Most of these were the result of mishandling industrial radioisotope sources or through inadvertent exposure of workers to industrial x-rays. Often the accidents took place because unsuspecting people – including children – picked up a curious metal object and took it home, only to become exposed with their families to the radiation emitted from the metal-encapsulated source.

Between 300 and 500 people were irradiated in Ciudad Juarez, Mexico, in 1983, when an abandoned cobalt-60 source found its way into a shipment of scrap metal: the delivery truck that carried it, the roadsides, and the steel that was made from the scrap were all contaminated. The next year an entire family of eight in Mohammedia, Morocco, died after a passer-by picked up an iridium-192 source used in construction and took it home. And in 1987 in Goiania, Brazil, some 240 people were contaminated when a caesium-137 source was taken home and dismantled; 54 were taken to hospital, and four died.

Accidents have also occurred in nuclear installations. Prior to Chernobyl, the two worst accidents happened within a fortnight of each other, in the autumn of 1957. Both were at military plants where designs,

MAN-MADE SOURCES

conditions and standards were very different from those at today's civil installations. On 29 September, a chemical explosion in a concrete tank containing nuclear waste in the southern Urals in the Soviet Union scattered some 74 quadrillion becquerel of radioactive materials over the provinces of Chelyabinsk, Sverdlovsk and Tyumensk; more than 10,000 people were evacuated during the next 18 months. On 7 October, a maintenance operation was started on the Windscale number one plutonium production reactor in Cumbria in northwest England. A fire was detected on 10 October and finally extinguished on 12 October, after a release of radioactive materials that led to an estimated collective dose commitment of 1300 man-sievert. The accident received massive media coverage at the time, with a series of press conferences and reports to Parliament. Some of the details, however, did not emerge till much later.

The only serious accident to a civil installation before Chernobyl was at the Three Mile Island power station in Pennsylvania in 1979. There, the built-in protective features of the plant, which were not present at either of the military installations, prevented the release of large amounts of radioactive materials. But all these events were dwarfed by what happened at Chernobyl.

At 1.23 on the morning of 26 April 1986, there was a major accident in the fourth unit of the Chernobyl power station in the Ukraine, about 100 kilometres from Kiev. It caused extensive local contamination and spread radioactive materials over the western Soviet Union and Europe, and, to a lesser extent, throughout the rest of the northern hemisphere. Governments and scientists were surprised by the way in which a single accident could have such a widespread impact.

The accident took place as the three-year-old RMBK-1000 reactor was undergoing a routine shutdown. A test was being carried out to see how long the steam turbines could generate electricity in the event of a blackout. The test procedures were themselves unsafe, and the operators repeatedly violated safety rules, putting the reactor into a dangerous condition. Eventually the operators, deliberately and against the rules, withdrew most

MAN-MADE SOURCES

of the control rods from the reactor core and switched off some important safety systems.

As the reactor began to run out of control, the operators made a vain attempt to prevent disaster. But it was too late. The power surged to 100 times its normal level in just four seconds. Part of the fuel shattered, and set off a steam explosion which lifted the 1000 tonne lid off the reactor. Two or three seconds later another explosion blew parts of the reactor right out of the building. Air rushed in, and the graphite blocks in the reactor core caught fire.

Vast quantities of radioactive materials were released over the next 10 days – one quarter of them during the first day of the accident. For five days the emissions fell as helicopters dropped boron carbide, dolomite, clay and lead onto the core, and then started rising rapidly, as the remaining fuel in the damaged core heated up to 2000 degrees centigrade. Between 1 and 5 May, they rose threefold until they stood at two-thirds of the levels released on the first catastrophic day. It was only on 6 May that they were finally brought under control.

Over those 10 days the winds shifted, dispersing clouds of contaminated air all over Europe. The force of the initial explosions and the intensity of the fire thrust radioactive materials 1500 metres into the air and southeasterly winds carried them over the western Soviet Union to Finland and Sweden, arriving on 27 April. A second contaminated cloud, blown by more easterly winds, drifted over eastern and central Europe reaching Switzerland and northern Italy on 30 April; southerly winds then carried radioactive materials northwards over France, Belgium, the Netherlands and the United Kingdom over the next two days. A third cloud, drifting southwards from Chernobyl over the southwestern Soviet Union, Romania, Yugoslavia and Bulgaria reached southern Greece on 3 May.

This is, inevitably, a highly simplified summary of a complex pattern of emissions and winds, which also brought radioactive materials to Spain, Israel, Kuwait and Turkey in early May. Indeed, by the time the releases were brought under control on 6 May, long range atmospheric transport had carried activity emitted from the damaged core throughout the northern hemisphere, where 88% of the world's people live; for example, it arrived in Japan on 2 May, China on 4 May, India on 5 May, and both western and eastern Canada and the United States over 5 to 6 May. Naturally, as the radioactive material spread it became increasingly thinly scattered over distant regions. No radioactive materials from the accident appear to have reached the southern hemisphere; there is little transfer of air masses across the Equator.

The pattern of fall-out across the Soviet Union and Europe was even more complicated. Radioactive materials are largely brought to earth by rainfall, and this was sporadic throughout the continent at the time. An area became contaminated if it happened to rain while the pollution from Chernobyl was passing overhead. If the weather stayed dry while the cloud

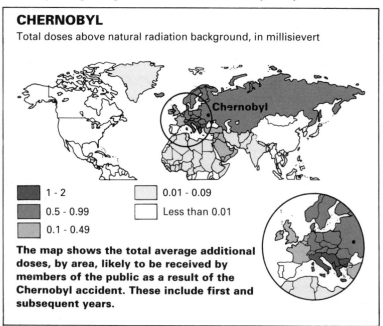

CHERNOBYL

Total doses above natural radiation background, in millisievert

Chernobyl

1 - 2	0.01 - 0.09
0.5 - 0.99	Less than 0.01
0.1 - 0.49	

The map shows the total average additional doses, by area, likely to be received by members of the public as a result of the Chernobyl accident. These include first and subsequent years.

MAN-MADE SOURCES

---

was passing, or it rained before or after the critical period, the area largely escaped.

Part of Sweden, north of Stockholm, was particularly unlucky, receiving the highest deposition of caesium-137 anywhere outside the Soviet Union. Other areas to the east of the country were also badly affected, the south and west were contaminated to a much lesser extent, and the north of the country escaped. Particularly high levels of fall-out from Chernobyl were also recorded in southern Bavaria and south Switzerland, and in the Austrian provinces of Salzburg, Carinthia and Upper Austria.

Using estimates of the average amounts of caesium-137 deposited all over the northern hemisphere, UNSCEAR has calculated that about 70 quadrillion becquerel of the radionuclide were emitted from Chernobyl, about a quarter of the amount in the reactor core when the accident occurred. This compares with an estimate of 38 quadrillion becquerel by Soviet scientists from local measurements. Given the magnitude of the uncertainties in each estimate, they agree reasonably well. About 42% of this was deposited in the Soviet Union, 37% in Europe, 6% in the oceans and the rest scattered over the land masses of the rest of the northern hemisphere. Similarly, UNSCEAR estimated that 35 quadrillion becquerel of caesium-134 and 330 quadrillion becquerel of iodine-131 may have been released. These three radionuclides are the main contributors to doses as a result of the accident.

People have received doses of radiation from the accident in four ways: they were irradiated directly by the cloud as it passed by; they breathed in contaminated air; they received external doses from ground affected by fall-out; and they consumed contaminated food. UNSCEAR has worked out rough estimates of the doses received from each of these pathways, using such information as is available.

Direct irradiation from the brief passage of the cloud is much the least important; everywhere it contributes less than 1% of the effective dose commitment received in the first year after the accident. Breathing in the radioactive materials is also a relatively minor component of the total dose in most areas. Overall, it contributes an average of 5% to the first-year committed effective doses: but this varies enormously in different places, ranging from a contribution of 0.1% in Ireland to 22% in Turkey.

External doses from ground affected by fall-out and internal doses from contaminated food are much more important in the short term, and account for almost all the long-term dose. Several short-lived radionuclides, including iodine-131, played an important part in the external irradiation for the first month after deposition, while ruthenium-103 and 106 made contributions for several months. But since then the only significant sources have been caesium-134 and 137. Caesium-134 will continue to give elevated doses for years, and caesium-137 for decades. But the doses will vary greatly, depending on the amount of fall-out that occurred in specific regions at the time.

Food contamination is even more variable, because it depends not just on whether there was rain when the Chernobyl cloud passed over, but on the agricultural season and practices in the region. Concentrations of iodine-131 in milk in Sweden, for example, were kept rather low because the accident took place just before cows were due to go out to pasture for the summer. They were kept indoors for some days longer than usual, allowing short-lived iodine-131 to decay and keeping doses lower than in countries where cattle were already grazing in pastures which became contaminated. Similarly, leafy vegetables picked up less of the radionuclide in Scandinavia than in southern Europe, because the growing season was less advanced. So doses from iodine-131 were less than 4% of the total in Scandinavia, compared with 20% in some more southerly countries.

Caesium-134 and 137 became the dominant radionuclides as the short lived iodine-131 decayed, and they accounted for more than half of the first-year dose from contaminated foodstuffs in most countries. Some foods contained particularly high levels, including mushrooms in Germany, freshwater fish in Sweden, and reindeer in Scandinavia. These foods are eaten in small amounts by many people, and in large amounts by relatively few; thus their contamination can have serious local effects – as in the

MAN-MADE SOURCES

disruption of the lives of Lapps dependent on reindeer – but makes a relatively small overall contribution to collective doses. Sheep and goats' milk in Greece contained far higher levels of iodine-131 than cows' milk, because of their different metabolism and feeding habits.

In all, contaminated food contributed most of the total effective dose commitment over the first year, and increased in proportion towards the south. Its contribution ranged from 69% in Scandinavia to 86% in southern countries like Greece, compared with 27% and 11% respectively for external radiation. As time goes by, however, external radiation becomes increasingly important, and UNSCEAR expects it to provide rather more than half of the full effective dose commitments in all but the southern countries. At the same time caesium-137 will become the dominant radionuclide of concern. Most of the effective dose commitment will be delivered within 30 years of the accident, 30% of it was received in the first year.

Emergency precautionary measures in the Soviet Union and Europe reduced the potential dose from the accident. Some 115,000 people were evacuated from a 30 kilometre radius around the reactor after the accident, tens of thousands of cattle were removed from the area and the consumption of locally produced milk and other foods was banned over a large area. Potassium iodide was given to 5.4 million people in the Soviet Union as a protection against the uptake of iodine-131. As a result, thyroid doses were reduced by 80 to 90% in the most contaminated region of the Soviet Union. Such countermeasures as the banning of contaminated foods were reported to have reduced doses of caesium-137 by 20 to 80% in the Soviet Union, by between 30 and 50% in Austria, Germany and Norway – and somewhat less in other countries.

UNSCEAR has mainly been concerned to estimate the overall impact of the accident over the entire globe, leaving individual national and local assessments to the countries concerned; its local estimates may, therefore, lack precision. It has instead calculated first-year committed doses and effective dose commitments for wider areas. Averaging out over large areas and many people inevitably conceals big variations between localities and individuals.

As a result, these first-year dose estimates show that the Soviet Union's average effective dose, at 0.82 millisievert per person, is lower than the 1.2 millisievert calculated for southeastern Europe (Bulgaria, Greece, Italy and Yugoslavia), than the 0.97 millisievert calculated for Scandinavia and than the 0.94 millisievert estimated for central Europe. This is because the Soviet Union's figure inevitably represents the dose averaged over the whole of that vast country, most of which was scarcely affected by the accident. More specifically, the Byelorussian SSR received the highest average first-year effective dose commitment – two millisievert, about the same as received annually from natural radiation. Subregions in Romania and Switzerland received one to two millisievert, and parts of Austria, Bulgaria, Germany and Yugoslavia received 0.5 to one millisievert.

In all, UNSCEAR estimated in 1988 that the accident resulted in a total collective effective dose commitment of 600,000 man-sievert; 53% of it has been, or will be, experienced in European countries, 36% in the Soviet Union, 8% in Asia, 2% in Africa and 0.3% in North, Central and South America. This dose is not very great compared with exposures to natural radiation, if averaged out over entire continents or the world as a whole; but of course the local and regional impact could be very great. The individual doses to the most affected populations in the local regions near the accident site in the Soviet Union – and their effects – are being evaluated in more detail by Soviet scientists, with reviews by international experts.

OCCUPATIONAL EXPOSURES

Accidents apart, the people who get the largest doses of radiation from the nuclear power industry are the several hundred thousand people who work in it around the world. As in almost all industries, the biggest regular exposures are occupational.

Difficulties bedevil attempts to assess occupational doses; conditions vary widely and there is not enough information. Exposures inside nuclear

MAN-MADE SOURCES

facilities differ just as emissions do; some of the various devices used to monitor radiation doses are designed to ensure that workers are not exposed to undue levels but they do not provide the kind of information required for detailed dose assessments. More individual monitoring is now taking place, however, and better data are being accumulated.

Estimates for uranium mines and mills suggest that their workers receive averages of 0.7 man-sievert of radiation for every gigawatt year of electrical energy eventually generated from their production. Mines are responsible for virtually all this dose, and, naturally, underground mines generally subject the people who work in them to greater doses than do open-cast ones. Fuel manufacturing facilities produce a collective equivalent dose of about 0.5 man-sievert per gigawatt year.

These figures conceal a wide variety of doses, and such variations are even more marked in nuclear reactors. Measurements at pressurized heavy water reactors, for example, show that collective doses per gigawatt year of electricity have varied a hundredfold. By and large, newer power stations produce lower doses than older ones. On average, reactors seem to produce annual collective effective doses of 10 man-sievert per gigawatt year.

Large numbers of workers at both the Sellafield and La Hague reprocessing plants are occupationally exposed – 5600 at Sellafield and 3700 at La Hague in 1985. Average individual doses fell at both plants during the 1980s. At Sellafield, the average in 1980 was 8.2 millisievert, in 1985, 5.6 millisievert and in 1989, 2.9 millisievert. At La Hague, averages doses between 1973 and 1977 were between four and five millisievert, in 1985 they were just over two millisievert. The collective dose per unit of electricity generated by the reprocessed fuel is much higher at Sellafield than at La Hague, mainly because of the relatively low energy per tonne of the Magnox fuel that is reprocessed at Sellafield compared with the predominately oxide fuel that is reprocessed at La Hague. The 1985 Sellafield figure of 18.9 man-sievert per gigawatt year was more than 20 times the La Hague level. The new reprocessing plant being built at Sellafield will reprocess oxide fuel and is likely to give much lower doses,

MAN-MADE SOURCES

and so UNSCEAR estimates that five man-sievert per gigawatt year may be a realistic future global figure. As only 5% of the world's fuel is reprocessed, there is a collective dose of 0.25 man-sievert per gigawatt year worldwide.

Workers engaged in nuclear research and development receive doses that vary particularly widely between plants and countries. Collective doses per unit of electrical energy produced differ tenfold from country to country; they are, for example, low in Japan and Switzerland, and high in the United Kingdom. A realistic worldwide figure for these workers might be five man-sievert per gigawatt year. Meanwhile the transport of radioactive materials adds a dose of 0.2 man-sievert per gigawatt year.

These estimates add up to a rough total annual collective equivalent dose of about 12 man-sievert for every gigawatt year of electricity generated – or a total of just over 2000 man-sievert in 1985. This is about 0.02% of the corresponding dose from natural sources.

This figure, which extends the occupational doses over the entire population obscures the fact that some radiation workers receive greater doses from their work than from natural sources. Underground uranium miners have usually received the highest average doses, over six times the average from natural sources. Sellafield workers in 1985 received more than twice the level people normally get from natural sources. Open-cast miners and workers at PWR, BWR and PHWR power stations receive rather less, but only workers at La Hague and in gas cooled reactors and fuel fabrication plants receive average additional doses of about the same magnitude as the average from natural radiation. And these average occupational doses conceal wide individual variations.

Of course, it is not only workers in the nuclear industry who receive occupational doses of man-made radiation. Medical and general industrial workers are also exposed. Exposures of medical personnel vary from country to country; averages range from 0.1 to three millisievert a year. Large numbers of workers are involved (there are at least 100,000 in the United States alone; more in Japan and Germany). Annual average doses for dentists are somewhat lower. Overall, it is estimated that the exposure

---

of medical personnel engaged in radiological work contributed about one man-sievert per million people to the collective effective dose in countries with a high standard of medical care. Poor conditions ensure that the collective dose in developing countries is probably about the same, even though there is far less radiological work. Occupational doses from radiotherapy are higher than from x-ray diagnosis, averaging from one to three man-sievert a year.

DOSES TO NUCLEAR REACTOR WORKERS

BWR } PWR }	13
GCR	5
PHWR	4
LWGR	2

man Sv per gigawatt year

Average doses to workers at different reactor types during 1980 to 1984, expressed in terms of collective dose per gigawatt year of electricity generated.

The use of radiation in general industry may produce an annual collective dose of about another 0.5 man-sievert per million population in industrialized countries. Many thousands of workers seem to be exposed, and permitted exposures are officially controlled; but little is known about the doses they actually receive, because records are not held centrally and therefore it is difficult to collect data. The relatively small numbers who use radioactive materials for making products luminous receive high annual average doses.

MAN-MADE SOURCES

Industrial radiographers use radiation under what are often rather primitive conditions on building sites and the like. Exposures among industrial radiographers vary widely depending on their workload and the techniques they use. Some are among the most highly exposed of all workers, and, as a group, industrial radiographers are the most likely to suffer from accidental overexposures to radiation.

Some workers are exposed to higher doses of natural radiation than usual by the nature of their work. Aircrew form the largest group: the altitude at which they work increases their exposure to cosmic rays. Some 70,000 aircrew in the United States, and 20,000 in the United Kingdom receive an average of between one and two millisievert extra a year.

Far beneath them, coal and metal miners also receive enhanced doses. These are highly variable, but – in some forms of underground mining, other than coal mining – can rival the higher exposures found in uranium mines. Workers at radon spas, where people go for supposedly beneficial treatment, can receive very high doses, sometimes exceeding 300 millisievert a year – six times the internationally recommended exposure limit in a single year for nuclear workers.

MISCELLANEOUS SOURCES

Finally, some common consumer products contain materials which expose a generally unaware public to radiation.

Luminous watches and clocks provide much the biggest worldwide dose. They have an annual impact four times as great as environmental releases from nuclear energy, and give rise to the same collective equivalent dose as from air travel or from occupational exposures in the nuclear industry – 2000 man-sievert .

Watches used to be luminized with radium. This exposes the whole body of the owner to penetrating radiation – though the dose is 10,000 times greater one centimetre from the dial than it is one metre away. It is now tending to be replaced by tritium or promethium-147, which give much smaller doses. Yet by the end of the 1970s, 800,000 watches containing

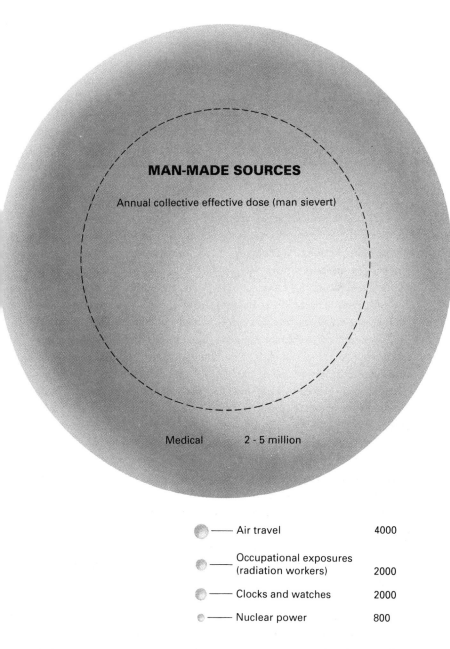

MAN-MADE SOURCES

Annual collective effective dose (man sievert)

Medical   2 - 5 million

● —— Air travel   4000

● —— Occupational exposures
        (radiation workers)   2000

● —— Clocks and watches   2000

● —— Nuclear power   800

Comparison of annual collective doses from man-made sources of radiation.

MAN-MADE SOURCES

radium were still in use in the United Kingdom. International standards for radium in watches were published in 1967, but many watches still in use may predate them. Radionuclides are also used to illuminate exit signs, compasses, gun sights, telephone dials, and many other devices.

Anti-static brushes using alpha particles are sold in the United States to remove dust from gramophone records and photographic equipment. In 1975, the United Kingdom's National Radiological Protection Board (NRPB) found these could be dangerous in certain circumstances.

Many smoke detectors also use alpha radiation. More than 26 million of them, incorporating americium-241, had been installed in the United States by the end of the 1970s, but they only emit tiny doses in normal use. Radionuclides are also used in starters for fluorescent tube lights and some electrical appliances. Nearly a hundred million such products were in use in Germany alone in the mid 1970s. Unless they are broken, they do not cause significant doses.

Thorium is used in some specially thin optical lenses, and can deliver substantial doses to the lens of the eye. Uranium is commonly used in false teeth to make them shine, and can irradiate the tissues of the mouth. The United Kingom's NRPB has recommended that its use be discontinued; and the United States and Germany, which make most dental porcelain, limit concentrations. Both these uses are purely for aesthetic reasons, and so the resulting exposures are entirely unjustified.

X-rays are produced inside colour televisions, but modern sets emit only negligible amounts as long as they are used normally and serviced appropriately. X-ray machines used for screening baggage give air travellers only minute doses each trip. More seriously, disturbing surveys in the United States and Canada in the early 1970s showed that many secondary schools were using x-ray tubes that could emit high doses – and that most teachers demonstrating them had little or no knowledge of radiation protection.

CHAPTER FIVE

EFFECTS ON PEOPLE

Radiation, by its very nature, is harmful to life. At low doses, it can start off only partially understood chains of events which lead to cancer or genetic damage, and it can kill cells. Cell killing is only important at high doses, when the body cannot replace the dead cells quickly enough. Cancer and genetic damage may be caused at any dose level.

The damage done by high doses normally becomes evident within hours or days. Cancers, however, take many years – usually decades – to emerge. And, by definition, the hereditary malformations and diseases caused by genetic damage take generations to show; it is the children, grandchildren, or remoter descendants of the people originally irradiated who will be affected.

Whereas it is usually quite easy to identify the early, acute effects of high doses, it is almost always extremely hard to pin down these "late" effects from low doses. This is partly because you have to wait much longer for them to become evident. Even then it is hard to apportion blame because both cancer and genetic damage are not specific to radiation but have many other causes.

Radiation doses have to reach a certain level to produce acute injury – but not to cause cancer or genetic damage. In theory, at least, just the smallest dose can be sufficient. So no level of exposure to radiation can be described as safe. Yet, at the same time, no level is uniformly dangerous. Even at quite high doses not everyone is affected; the body's repair mechanisms usually offset the damage that is done. Similarly, someone exposed to a dose of radiation is by no means fated to develop cancer or sustain genetic damage; but he is at greater risk than if he had not been irradiated. And the size of the risk will increase with the size of the dose.

UNSCEAR tries to work out, as reliably as possible, just what extra risks people face from different doses of radiation. Probably more research has been carried out on the effects of radiation than on any similar hazard. But the longer-term the effect, and the lower the dose, the less information there is.

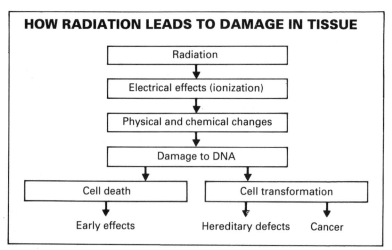

HOW RADIATION LEADS TO DAMAGE IN TISSUE

Radiation
↓
Electrical effects (ionization)
↓
Physical and chemical changes
↓
Damage to DNA

Cell death | Cell transformation

Early effects | Hereditary defects | Cancer

There are several complex stages between radiation hitting a cell and its final effects.

EARLY EFFECTS

It is important to study the effects in man in the first two to three months following doses of about one gray or more of x-ray or gamma radiation to the whole body because of the persistent possibility that people will become exposed to high doses as a result of radiation accidents or nuclear war.

Reliable information on the subject is very limited; such data as are available come from the effects of the Second World War A-bombs on the people of Hiroshima and Nagasaki, experience with patients given whole-body irradiation to treat cancer or prepare them for organ transplants, and from accidental exposures.

The Chernobyl accident has added to our understanding of the acute effects of high whole-body doses and will enhance our knowledge further when all the information collected has been fully analyzed. In all, 237 people suffered from radiation sickness as a result of the accident and 115 people received doses above one gray. Within three months of the accident

EFFECTS ON PEOPLE

28 members of the reactor's operating staff and fire fighting crew had died from their exposure to radiation; another two deaths – one in the explosions themselves and one from ordinary heat burns – were unconnected with radiation. There is information on the size of the doses and the duration of exposure that the victims received and exhaustive data on what happened to them and what treatment they underwent.

Radiation sickness is the first effect of high, whole-body doses. Symptoms include loss of appetite, nausea, vomiting, diarrhea, intestinal cramps, salivation, dehydration, fatigue, apathy, listlessness, sweating, fever, headache and low blood pressure. Any one exposed to a very high dose, of several tens of gray, will begin to show all these symptoms within five to 15 minutes. Lower doses delay the onset of sickness and produce less severe symptoms; about half of those who receive doses of two gray suffer vomiting after about three hours, and the symptom is rare after doses below one gray.

In many cases radiation sickness is the prelude to a painful death. Generally speaking, doses higher than 50 gray damage the central nervous system so badly that death occurs within a few days. At doses of 10 to 50 gray, the victim may escape this fate only to die from gastrointestinal damage between one and two weeks later. Lower doses may avoid gastrointestinal injury or permit recovery from it – but still cause death after a month or two, mainly from damage to the red bone marrow – the tissue that forms blood.

The red bone marrow and the rest of the blood-forming system are affected by as little as 0.5 to one gray. Fortunately they also have a remarkable capacity for regeneration and, if the dose is not so great as to overwhelm them, can completely recover from these early effects, although they will always be at a higher risk of developing leukemia in later years. If only part of the body is irradiated, enough bone marrow will normally survive unimpaired to replace what is damaged. Animal experiments suggest the chances of people dying from a given dose can be reduced from 50% to zero, if only a tenth of the active bone marrow escapes irradiation.

EFFECTS ON PEOPLE

UNSCEAR has examined the evidence to try to work out the dose of radiation that will kill half the people exposed to it from bone marrow failure within 60 days. This information is vital in planning for the effects of nuclear war, accidents or other emergencies because the authorities need to know roughly how many casualties to expect. Evidence from Hiroshima and Nagasaki suggests that half of those exposed to about three gray died within this time period and studies of seriously ill cancer patients yield about the same result. But the experience of the Chernobyl victims and of relatively healthy cancer patients suggest that more than half of those affected at this dose level survived if they received intensive treatment.

UNSCEAR has come to the conclusion that it is impossible to determine a single dose that will always have this effect on people; in reality, much may depend on the age and health of those irradiated and the treatment they receive. It suggests that a dose of about 2.5 gray, or higher, may be sufficient to kill half of a group of cancer patients or healthy people who receive little or no medical treatment after exposure, as in the devastation that followed the atomic bomb explosions. A dose of three gray, however, may kill few healthy humans and it may take five gray, or approaching it, to prove fatal for half a group of healthy people who receive good medical care, such as the Chernobyl victims. Similarly, a dose of six or seven gray would kill virtually all the healthy people exposed to it, while five to six gray would have the same effect on cancer patients.

10,000 mSv

EFFECTS ON PEOPLE

EFFECTS OF RADIATION
millisievert

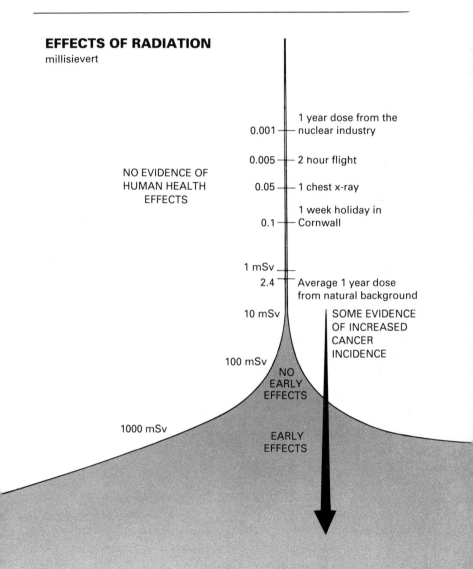

NO EVIDENCE OF
HUMAN HEALTH
EFFECTS

0.001 — 1 year dose from the
nuclear industry

0.005 — 2 hour flight

0.05 — 1 chest x-ray

0.1 — 1 week holiday in
Cornwall

1 mSv

2.4 — Average 1 year dose
from natural background

10 mSv

SOME EVIDENCE
OF INCREASED
CANCER
INCIDENCE

100 mSv

NO
EARLY
EFFECTS

1000 mSv

EARLY
EFFECTS

FATAL DOSE

EFFECTS ON PEOPLE

DELAYED EFFECTS
Cancer

Cancer is much the most important effect of low level radiation – at least as far as those actually exposed are concerned. It is also the greatest cause of death in industrialized countries after cardiovascular disease, responsible for about 20 to 25% of all fatalities. It has been estimated that some 85 to 90%, perhaps even more, of all cancers are due to environmental factors – including exposures to environmental carcinogens, diet, smoking and other personal habits.

No-one knows how great radiation's contribution is to this toll. No single type of cancer is uniquely caused by exposure to radiation: indeed most, perhaps all, common cancers can result from it, though with varying degrees of probability. For many years it was thought that some human organs were relatively insusceptible, but it now appears that most, and probably all, organs are vulnerable to some extent. But it is impossible to distinguish radiation-induced tumours from those arising from many other causes. Because radiation leaves no particular trademark of damage, appearing to cause the same cellular anomalies as other carcinogens, it is rarely, if ever, possible to state categorically that radiation has – or has not – caused a specific cancer.

Even after many decades of study there are many fundamental uncertainties. The development of a cancer seems to be a complex process, comprising a number of stages. Some initiating phenomenon, most probably affecting a single cell, appears to start the process, but a series of other events seem to be necessary before the cell becomes malignant and the tumour develops. Nobody knows how the process works or what stage or stages can be affected by radiation. Cancers only become evident long after the first damage is done, following a period of latency. Leukemias and bone cancers first appear at least two to five years after exposure to radiation, while solid tumours are not expressed until the passage of at least 10 years, often several decades.

Nevertheless, it is important to try to estimate the risks of contracting

EFFECTS ON PEOPLE

cancer from particular doses of radiation in order to provide a sound scientific basis for setting exposure limits. There is a wealth of experimental information from animal tests, but, while it helps, it cannot substitute for evidence of what happens to people. Much effort is expended in examining the fate of people who have actually been exposed to doses of radiation in the past, and establishing whether they are more likely to contract cancer than those who have not been irradiated – and by how much. UNSCEAR surveys research on people who have received radiation therapy, those who have been exposed to radiation in their jobs, people contaminated by fall-out from bomb tests, and – above all – those who were irradiated by, but survived, the A-bomb explosions at Hiroshima and Nagasaki in 1945.

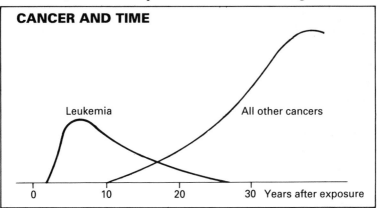

Such studies are beset with difficulties. The evidence must fulfil a whole set of conditions if valid estimates of risks are to be made – and none of the research adequately meets them all. There is rarely sufficient information on what dose of radiation was received by each individual. The studies have not yet gone on long enough for all the cancers to emerge after their latency periods: research should continue until all the irradiated people have died, but the studies are often abandoned too early. Follow-up diagnoses are often not good enough to catch all the cancers. The irradiated people are frequently not typical of the general population in their state of

---

health, in their exposure to carcinogenic agents other than radiation or in their breakdown by age, sex, or socioeconomic status. The "control" population – which should be similar in every relevant way to the people being studied, except for the fact that they have not been irradiated – is seldom adequate to ensure that good enough comparisons can be made.

The most valuable studies are those that allow estimates of the effects of radiation on a large variety of parts of the body. Only three studies provide enough information to do this.These are the studies of 76,000 A-bomb survivors in Japan, of 14,000 Britons irradiated for the treatment of ankylosing spondylitis, and of an international collection of 83,000 women given radiotherapy for cervical cancer. All cover a large sample of people who received some exposure over many parts of the body and who were followed up over reasonably long, if still inadequate, periods. But they have major drawbacks. The ankylosing spondylitis and cervical cancer patients were already sick when irradiated (and had already been receiving medication) and were thus not representative of the general population, and the cancer patients may well already have been particularly susceptible to the disease. Furthermore, more than four-fifths of the ankylosing spondylitis patients were men, while, naturally, all the cervical cancer patients were women. Neither includes enough people under the age of 25, and neither can provide individual dose estimates for most of the patients.

The Japanese data are much the best because a large number of people, largely representative of the general population, received a wide variety of doses spread fairly evenly over the body. It has long been the single most important source of information, and UNSCEAR has used it as the main source of risk estimates, though it is checked against many other studies. But it has drawbacks, too. Estimates of the doses received by the A-bomb survivors have had to be revised, and, even after this has been done, the exposures received by almost a fifth of them still cannot be computed. As in the other main studies, not enough time has yet elapsed to follow the entire population through to death; indeed the youngest children at the time of the bombings are only now entering the key stage of their adult lives when cancer prevalence increases.

More fundamentally still, almost all the data are based on the study of people whose tissues have received quite high doses of radiation, one gray or more, either as a single dose or over relatively short periods. There is scant information on the effects of receiving low doses for a long time: there are just a few studies on the effects of the range of doses normally received by workers with radiation, and there is no direct information at all about the consequences of exposures routinely received by the general public. So there is no alternative to trying to derive estimates of risks at low

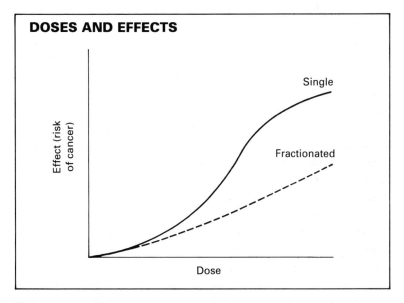

DOSES AND EFFECTS

Risk of cancer increases with increasing dose. Evidence of harm is only available at high doses and high dose rates. Low doses are less harmful (per unit dose) than high doses. Low dose rates (a given dose spread over a long period – or fractionated) are less harmful than high dose rates (the same dose given in a short time). This applies to gamma and beta radiation. For alpha radiation, the effect is directly proportional to the dose at all dose rates.

73

EFFECTS ON PEOPLE

doses from what little is known about hazards at high ones.

To do so, UNSCEAR – like other bodies working in the field – makes two basic assumptions, which broadly fit what evidence there is. The first is that there is no threshold at which there is no risk of cancer. Any dose, however small, increases the chances that the person who receives it will get cancer – and every additional dose will increase those chances further. The second assumption is that the risk increases in direct proportion to the dose. The relationship between dose and risk is approximately linear over a limited range of doses. In other words, over that range, doubling the dose would double the risk. The risk at low doses and dose rates, however, is lower than would be calculated by a linear extrapolation of the risk at high doses and dose rates, by a factor that UNSCEAR believes should lie between two and 10.

Over the last 30 years, UNSCEAR has revised its estimates of cancer risks upwards on several occasions, as more evidence became available from Hiroshima and Nagasaki and other studies and as understanding of the data increased. The most recent of these revisions took place in its latest report, in 1988, and followed a complete re-evaluation of the doses received by the A-bomb victims. This reassessment, initiated by the governments of Japan and the United States and culminating in 1986, disclosed that doses from the especially damaging neutron radiation were substantially lower than had previously been thought, and other revisions also had to be made. It appears that the cancers that have materialized among the A-bomb survivors resulted from lower doses than had been supposed, and therefore the risk per unit of dose must be greater than had been believed. At the same time, more cancers kept emerging in the survivors as time went on. This also supported an upward revision of the risk estimates. Besides, calculations of the doses received by the ankylosing spondylitis patients have also been revised, and further information on the number of cancer deaths in various studies have supported an increased risk.

In 1977, UNSCEAR estimated that about 25 people out of every 1000 would die of cancer for every gray they received, at doses of one to several gray. After the revision of doses, UNSCEAR produced new estimates for its 1988 report. It now calculates that between 40 and 110 people out of every thousand in a population of all ages and both sexes exposed to a dose of one gray will contract fatal cancer. It also calculates that the same dose will deprive the same population of a total of 950 to 1400 years of life due to premature death from the disease. It is important to note that these figures and those in the following paragraphs do not include an allowance for the reduction of risks at low doses and dose rates.

Two other factors contributed to this marked revision: the use of a new way of calculating risk, and new information on the particular vulnerability of children.

Since none of the large studies has yet been able to follow the irradiated populations through until everyone has died, UNSCEAR still has to compute the risk of getting cancer over entire lifetimes from the partial data that are available. It reached its 1977 estimate by means of the "additive" or "absolute" risk model, which assumes that (once the minimum latency period has run its course) the extra risk of an irradiated person getting cancer depends only on the dose received. But in 1988 it also used the "multiplicative" or "relative" risk model, which assumes that (again, once the minimum latency period has passed) the extra risk also increases with age; this naturally produces higher estimates than the additive model, but evidence from the Japanese research and other studies suggests that it fits the data better. The risk estimate in UNSCEAR's 1988 report is therefore a combination of calculations using both models. The additive model projected 40 to 50 cancer deaths per 1000 people who received doses of a single gray, the multiplicative model projected 70 to 110 fatalities: the latter, higher figures, appear on present evidence to be the more likely.

UNSCEAR is more precise when calculating the effects on adults alone; one gray, it estimates, will kill between 50 and 60 people in every 1000 people over age 25. The consequences for young people are much less well known, but are almost certainly much greater. Tissues are more

EFFECTS ON PEOPLE

susceptible to the effects of radiation when cells are proliferating, so children are particularly vulnerable as they grow and develop. Their youth also gives them more time to develop cancers with long latency periods. Yet hard information is sparse.

Evidence of the effects of the Hiroshima and Nagasaki bombing on children is far from complete because they have not yet reached the age at which many of the cancers appear. The best data are on leukemia; its brief latency period is even shorter in children. Young people under 20 appear to be about twice as likely to develop cancer as adults. Children under 10 are particularly susceptible; the multiplicative model suggests that they are three to four times more likely to die of leukemia than adults. The Japanese and other studies have also shown that girls under 20 are about twice as likely to develop breast cancer as adults and those under 10 face a substantial relative risk. Indeed, people irradiated as children are more likely than adults to get most kinds of cancer after irradiation, but the disease may not emerge until late in their lives when they reach the ages at which the cancers normally become evident.

In all, radiation has been shown to increase significantly the likelihood of getting at least 11 different types of cancer – leukemia, multiple myeloma, and cancers of the breast, thyroid, lung, stomach, oesophagus, colon, ovary, urinary bladder and central nervous system (other than the brain). The breast, thyroid and bone marrow seem to be particularly susceptible. UNSCEAR estimates that leukemia accounts for between 10 to 25% of all deaths from radiation-induced cancer. Breast and thyroid cancers affect far more people than they kill because both can commonly be cured. Only half the people who get breast cancer – and only a tenth of those who get thyroid cancer – are likely to die of it. Lung cancer, however, is a sure killer and, partly in consequence, is a significant cause of death from radiation exposure. Multiple myeloma and cancers of the colon and ovary have been added to the list since UNSCEAR reported in 1977, as a result of new evidence from Japan and the revision of dose estimates. No clear and significant excesses of deaths from malignant lymphoma or cancers of the mouth, gall bladder, rectum, pancreas, uterus, prostate or small intestine have yet been observed, but they may become evident as the population ages.

For the first time, slight but statistically significant increases in death from several kinds of cancer have been found among A-bomb survivors who received doses as low as 0.2 to 0.5 gray. But there is still considerable debate over how much of a risk there is from low level radiation. More research is needed. Studies of people exposed to levels of radiation usually encountered in the workplace and the environment would be particularly helpful. Unfortunately the lower the exposure, the harder it is to do meaningful research. It is estimated, for example, that, unless UNSCEAR's estimates are substantially out, a study of all cancers in nuclear workers exposed to 0.01 gray a year would need to cover several million person-years to have any hope of coming up with a significant result. And studies of people exposed to environmental levels would be harder still.

There are some even more complex issues requiring research. In principle, for example, radiation may interact with other chemical and biological agents to increase cancer rates further. Clearly, this is a particularly important issue because radiation is ubiquitous and because there are so many factors in modern life that could interact with it. UNSCEAR has carried out a preliminary analysis of information on a large number of such factors. Several suspects have emerged, and there is strong evidence on tobacco smoke. Uranium miners seem to get cancer earlier if they smoke, but the studies are conflicting and the extent of the increased risk is unclear.

There have long been suggestions that exposure to radiation may accelerate the aging process and so shorten life. UNSCEAR has reviewed the data on this hypothesis, and has been unable to find enough evidence to substantiate it, either in man or animals, at least at moderate to low long-term exposures. Irradiated populations do have a shorter average life-span, but this seems to be entirely accounted for by the increased number of individuals contracting cancer.

EFFECTS ON PEOPLE

Genetic effects

The study of genetic effects caused by radiation is even more difficult than the study of cancer. This is partly because there is extremely little information on what genetic damage humans sustain through irradiation, partly because the full tally of hereditary conditions takes many generations to show, and partly because, like cancer, these defects would be quite indistinguishable from those occurring from other causes.

Hereditary defects range from mild afflictions like colour blindness to severely incapacitating conditions like Down's syndrome, Huntington's chorea, or severe malformations. About 6% of all babies born alive suffer from some congenital abnormality. Some 60% of people may suffer from conditions such as hypertension, diabetes, coronary heart disease, epilepsy and multiple sclerosis – which have a genetic component – predominantly in later life.

Many of the severely affected embryos and foetuses do not survive; it has been estimated that about half of all spontaneous abortions have an abnormal genetic constitution. Even if they do survive to birth, babies with hereditary defects are about five times more likely to die before their fifth birthday than normal children.

Genetic effects fall into two main categories; chromosome aberrations involving changes in the number or structure of chromosomes, and mutations of the genes themselves. The gene mutations split further into dominant mutations, (which show in the children of the people who first sustained them) and recessive mutations (which only show up when two people with the same mutated gene jointly conceive a child; and so may lie dormant for many generations, or for ever). Both classes of effects can cause hereditary disease in subsequent generations, but will not necessarily do so. UNSCEAR's estimates concentrate only on severe hereditary conditions.

Studies of children whose parents were irradiated by the Hiroshima and Nagasaki bombs have failed to find a statistically significant incidence of genetic effects. This does not mean that no damage has been sustained,

EFFECTS ON PEOPLE

but that none has been detected. More research is needed. An international collaborative programme is being started to study genetic effects in the children of cancer patients treated with radiation; another worthwhile study is following up people exposed to radiation from the Chernobyl accident – and their children.

There is evidence that people exposed to low doses suffer detectable chromosome damage in their blood cells. This has been shown at remarkably low levels of exposure in people living at Badgastein, Austria, and working in its supposedly therapeutic radioactive springs. Nuclear workers exposed to less than the internationally accepted maximum permissible level of radiation in the United Kingdom, Germany and the United States also exhibit chromosome damage. But the biological significance and health consequences of such damage have not been established. A study by the Medical Research Council in the United Kingdom concluded that the children of workers at the Sellafield reprocessing complex who received doses to the testes of 100 millisievert or more were more likely to develop leukemia; this finding has not been supported by further studies and more research is being carried out.

In the absence of adequate data, it is necessary to estimate the risks of hereditary defects in man on the basis of extensive tests on animals. UNSCEAR employs two methods of trying to assess the risk to man. One concentrates directly on determining how much damage is done by a given dose of radiation. The other tries to derive what doses are needed to double the number of offspring that would normally be born with hereditary defects of different types.

The first method estimates that one gray of low level radiation administered to males alone will cause between 1000 and 2000 severe mutations and 100 to 1500 severe effects due to chromosome aberrations in every million births. The figures for the irradiation of women are much more uncertain, but lower, as female germ cells are less sensitive to radiation; rough calculations suggest that they range from 0 to 900 per million births for mutations and from 0 to 500 for chromosome aberrations.

EFFECTS ON PEOPLE

The second method estimates that continuous irradiation of one gray per generation (about 30 years) will produce 2000 severe cases of genetic disease per million births in the children of those exposed. It also attempts to work out the total number of defects that will arise over all generations if the same rate of exposure continues. It reckons that ultimately 12,000 children out of every million will continue to be born with severe disease as a result.

This method attempts to include the effects of recessive mutations. Not much is known about them, and they are still a subject of debate; but it is thought that they will only make a minor contribution as the chances of two people with exactly the same kind of gene damage mating are small. Little is known about whether, and to what extent, radiation exposures increase the prevalence of complex conditions – such as hypertension, diabetes and coronary heart disease – which are determined not by a single gene, but by many acting together. UNSCEAR's estimates concentrate on

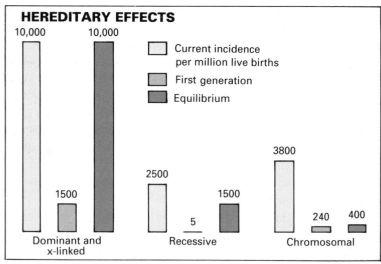

Incidence of severe genetic disease per million live births from a dose of one sievert per generation.

the effects on single genes because it is unable to quantify the contributions of such polygenic factors, and in the absence of further information it is not in a position to provide risk estimates for them.

Both methods of estimation are only able to address serious hereditary effects. The evidence strongly suggests that minor defects grossly outnumber serious ones, so much so that they could well cause more harm to the general population.

Attempts have been made to estimate the human impact of serious genetic defects. This involves assessing, and differentiating between, the harm from different genetic defects. For example, both Down's syndrome and Huntington's disease are serious genetic diseases – but they have a very different impact. Huntington's disease first strikes between the third and fifth decades of life and causes very serious, but gradual, degeneration of the central nervous system; Down's syndrome causes extremely serious problems from birth onwards. On this basis Down's syndrome might be thought to have the greater impact. On the other hand, sufferers from Huntington's disease often have children – and so pass on their condition to their progeny – unlike victims of Down's syndrome.

UNSCEAR is therefore attempting to evaluate the effects of genetic disease in terms of years of impaired and lost life, to try to give some idea of the impact of radiation-induced hereditary damage on its victims, their families, and society at large. Of course, even this would not make adequate allowance for the suffering of victims, and can make no allowance at all for such factors as the anguish of the parents of an affected child – these are impossible to quantify.

Effects on the unborn child

There is considerable concern about the effects of radiation on unborn children, exposed while still in the womb. The development of mammals in the womb falls roughly into three stages. The first lasts from conception to the point when the embryo settles into the wall of the womb, and covers the first two weeks of pregnancy in humans. The next, lasting from the

EFFECTS ON PEOPLE

second to eighth week in humans, covers the main period of the formation and development of the organs of the body: at the end of the eighth week, the human embryo – though weighing less than three grams – already possesses over 90% of the more than 4500 structures of the adult body. These continue to grow during the third period, which lasts until birth.

At each stage, radiation has a characteristic effect. Its main consequence in the first period is to kill the embryo in the womb. It is very hard to study what happens in this stage in human pregnancy and no new findings have been reported. There is, however, a great deal of new information from animal experiments, and this mainly confirms the special sensitivity of the early embryo to death from radiation.

During the next stage, the main danger is that radiation will lead to the growing organs becoming malformed, and perhaps cause death at around the time of birth. Animal experiments confirm that each structure – for example, the eyes, brain, or skeleton – is particularly susceptible to the induction of malformation if irradiated just at the point when it is developing. Evidence of such malformations in humans is rare. UNSCEAR believes, however, that this is not sufficient reason to discard the possibility that they do occur. It assumes that humans face the same risks as animals, and that, at worst, half of all foetuses receiving doses of a single gray in this stage of their development could become malformed.

The greatest damage done by radiation is to the central nervous system; this seems to occur after the eighth week, when the third stage of pregnancy begins. A great deal of progress has recently been made in understanding the effects of the Hiroshima and Nagasaki bombs on the brains of unborn children, and the revision of the doses has allowed important progress to be made on establishing the risks and consequences of irradiation in the womb. One study has found that 30 people out of about 1600 exposed before birth to radiation from the explosions are extremely mentally retarded; they cannot take care of themselves, carry out a simple conversation, perform simple calculations, or are completely unmanageable or have had to be committed to institutions. The highest IQ recorded among them is 68.

Foetuses aged eight to 15 weeks after conception were the most severely affected. UNSCEAR reckons that four out of every 10 receiving an acute dose of one gray at this stage will suffer extreme mental retardation as a result. Those aged 16 to 25 weeks were also damaged, though less frequently: it is estimated that one in every 10 exposed to one gray will be severely retarded. After 25 weeks the risk seems to be very low; no case of severe mental retardation has been reported in anyone irradiated after this point.

Every gray of dose received depresses IQ by up to 30 points, and it seems that lower doses may also have an effect in lowering intelligence. A dose of, say, a tenth of a gray would not cause a perfectly normal individual to become severely retarded, but the resulting shift downwards in expected intelligence could force some of those who would otherwise be at the lower level of the IQ spectrum across the boundary to clinical subnormality.

There has been fierce controversy for several years over whether radiation exposure in the womb can cause cancer later in life. Animal experiments have failed to show any particular sensitivity and the human data seem to be contradictory. Children who survived irradiation in the womb at Hiroshima and Nagasaki have so far shown no evidence that they are more likely to develop cancer, according to studies based on the old dose estimates. But two larger, independent studies, carried out in the United Kingdom and the United States on children exposed to much lower doses of medical radiation before birth, have consistently shown that they are about 50% more likely to get leukemia and other cancers before they reach their tenth birthday. These studies have been criticized because of various, possibly confounding and biasing, factors. Cause and effect have not yet been proved, but it would be unacceptable to neglect the evidence until a plausible explanation for it is found. UNSCEAR therefore assumes, as a matter of prudence, that radiation has caused the extra cancers.

UNSCEAR has tried to work out the overall risks to unborn children

EFFECTS ON PEOPLE

for a number of effects of irradiation – death, malformation, mental retardation, and cancer – put together. In all, it reckons that no more than two out of every 1000 live-born children, who have been exposed to the low dose of a hundredth of a gray in the womb, will be affected – compared with the 6% who develop the same effects naturally.

CHAPTER SIX

ACCEPTABILITY OF RISKS

Why is fear of radiation so widespread? If the assessments reported in this booklet are correct, low level radiation poses a relatively small public hazard.

Many people readily accept much greater hazards from, for example, smoking and driving. There seems, moreover, to be little public concern about natural radiation, which contributes about four-fifths of average annual effective dose. Few people, for example, seem to move from areas with high background radiation to places offering lower exposures so as to minimize their risk of getting cancer. There has, however, been growing concern about radon in houses. And the greatest source of unnecessary artificial doses – over-high exposures from medical x-rays – gets little public attention. Almost all apprehension is focused on nuclear power, which – so long as it operates normally – is one of the smallest contributors to the overall dose.

Scientists and administrators in many countries are often annoyed by what they see as public irrationality – and sometimes even suggest that it is aroused by agitators who want to undermine society itself. This is unwise, as the Royal Society in the United Kingdom has pointed out. The public attitude is not as irrational as it seems and may be well-founded.

One reason for the gap in perception between the majority of experts and a growing proportion of the public may stem from the very imprecision of assessments of the effects of some exposures. This booklet has repeatedly stressed the problems involved in collecting reliable information on some types of radiation exposure and assessing their effects. Determining the acceptability of risks is far harder still. Little is known about why people react to risks as they do. And the available methods for measuring the costs and benefits of hazardous undertakings are still very imprecise.

This chapter, unlike the preceding four, is not based on the reports of UNSCEAR, which has not yet addressed this subject, though it may be a topic for future consideration.

ACCEPTABILITY OF RISKS

As illustrated in the previous chapter, measurements of the cost of disability and disease are still crude. Normally, these try to quantify the effects of excess mortality only, often in financial terms; at best they attempt some rough assessment of life impairment from gross injury. They cannot effectively value the impact of lesser damage to the quality of life, let alone take account of human distress and frustrated prospects. But the public does take such factors into account, however instinctively.

It is often even harder to assess benefits than to determine costs. Furthermore, it is not sufficient to show that a hazardous process benefits society as a whole; the people most at risk want to be sure that the benefit

AVERAGE ANNUAL RISK OF DEATH IN THE UNITED KINGDOM FROM SOME COMMON CAUSES

Cause	Risk of death per year
Smoking 10 cigarettes a day*	1 in 200
Natural causes, 40 years old	1 in 700
Road accidents	1 in 10,000
Accidents at home	1 in 10,000
Accidents at work	1 in 50,000
Average dose from nuclear power	1 in 20 million

* The risk includes all adverse effects of smoking; for lung cancer, the risk is about halved.

AVERAGE ANNUAL RISK OF DEATH IN THE UNITED KINGDOM FROM ACCIDENTS IN VARIOUS INDUSTRIES

Industry	Risk of death per year
Sea fishing	1 in 500
Coal mining	1 in 7000
Construction	1 in 10,000
Metal manufacture	1 in 17,000
Radiation worker* (1 mSv per year, average)	1 in 25,000
Textiles	1 in 28,000
Food, drink and tobacco	1 in 45,000
Timber and furniture	1 in 100,000
Clothing and footwear	1 in 300,000

* The risk shown includes potential cancers due to occupational exposure.

ACCEPTABILITY OF RISKS

to them outweighs the hazard. In radiation therapy for cancer the chance of a cure usually far outweighs the risks of the high doses, and the people receiving the doses are those who stand to benefit from them. Unjustified exposures from medical x-ray examinations provide an equally straightforward equation: the patient is being exposed to extra risk for no extra benefit.

Environmental exposure to radiation from nuclear power, however, presents a much more difficult problem to resolve. In the first place, it is society as a whole that enjoys whatever benefits the energy provides; the people living near nuclear facilities, who shoulder almost all the risk, get only a small proportion of the benefit. Secondly, there is genuine doubt over whether nuclear energy does provide a net benefit over the use of other fuels – though burning fossil fuels has the great disadvantage of adding to global warming.

Then there is a substantial difference between voluntary and involuntary risks. Some people gladly embrace especially high risks for fun; they find that danger adds to the enjoyment of hang-gliding or ski-jumping, for example. Others cheerfully defy great hazards for altruistic purposes; people regularly risk their lives to save animals, even if they do not own them. Both smoking and driving involve taking voluntary risks, which is one reason why many people find them acceptable.

But whereas the freedom to risk one's life and health is a necessary part of liberty, the freedom to impose such risk on others is not – and public opinion is acutely aware of this. It consistently takes a harsher view of imposed or involuntary risks. When people feel impotent in the face of such a risk, and have no control over it or means of protecting themselves from it, they are even less tolerant. Radiation from the nuclear fuel cycle is seen by the public as embodying all these undesirable characteristics.

The case for nuclear power also suffers as a result of a basic moral dilemma. People doubt whether it is right to bequeath radioactive wastes, which will remain dangerous far into the future, to subsequent generations – particularly as their descendants will have no control over the problem

ACCEPTABILITY OF RISKS

left to them and share none of the benefits provided by nuclear power. The fact that the same arguments apply to the vastly greater quantities of non-radioactive toxic wastes produced by mankind does not affect this issue. Nuclear power also suffers from its association with the revulsion people feel for nuclear war.

Furthermore, people fear catastrophes, however infrequent, more than small dangers, however common. Quite correctly, much of the fear of nuclear power is of the consequences of an accident – whether at a reactor, reprocessing plant, or waste disposal facility – rather than the effects of routine releases of radiation. The Chernobyl accident has, understandably, greatly exacerbated these fears. UNSCEAR has not tried to assess the probabilities of accidents, and those studies that have done so have failed to provide wide public assurance.

Attitudes to risk are also affected by the extent to which they are known. On the one hand, some risks are scarcely known to the public at all, and thus, unfortunately receive little attention: this probably accounts for the lack of adequate concern about radon in houses in most countries and unnecessary exposure to x-rays. On the other hand, familiarity also leads to complacency towards certain risks. One recent study showed that well-known risks, such as from motorcycle riding, skiing, climbing, smoking – and even muggers and heroin – inspired little fear. Nuclear power, on the other hand, was both one of the least familiar and one of the most feared sources of risk; interestingly, it was far more feared than asbestos, which was judged to be better known.

Secrecy – particularly the half-kept secret – fuels fear, and there has been too much of it in the past. There have also been too many bland reassurances, and admonitions that the experts know best. But the reassurances have been found wanting, and the experts – though undoubtedly highly knowledgeable in their own fields – often do not take a wide enough view. There has been a serious and continuing loss of credibility.

The public needs to be involved far more in assessing the risks it is

ACCEPTABILITY OF RISKS

---

being asked to undertake, and in passing judgement on them. Unless it is, it will be increasingly unwilling to accept them. For this purpose it needs full, factual and unemotional information. This booklet has been an attempt to increase general understanding of radiation - its sources, effects and risks.